ENDOVAGINAL ULTRASOUND

ENDOVAGINAL ULTRASOUND

Steven R. Goldstein, M.D.

Department of Obstetrics and Gynecology
New York University School of Medicine
New York, New York

With Contributions by

Arthur C. Fleischer, M.D.

Lawrence Grunfeld, M.D.

Donna M. Kepple, R.T., R.D.M.S.

Rudy E. Sabbagha, M.D.

Benjamin Sandler, M.D.

Alan R. Liss, Inc., New York

To the memory of my father,
Joseph M. Goldstein,
who taught me the importance of
honesty and sensitivity.

Second Printing, April 1989

Library of Congress Cataloging-in-Publication Data

Goldstein, Steven R.
    Endovaginal ultrasound.

    Includes index.
    1. Ultrasonics in obstetrics. I. Title.
RG527.5.U48G64   1988   618.2'07'543   88-13051
ISBN 0-8451-4263-1

Cover: Endovaginal ultrasound at 8 weeks LMP. The embryo is just beginning to unfold. It is contained within the amnion, which has not yet fused with the chorion. The yolk sac is seen to be extra-amniotic.

Contents

Contributors

Arthur C. Fleischer, M.D.
Department of Radiology and Radiological Sciences, Section of Ultrasound, and Department of OB/GYN, Vanderbilt University Medical Center, Nashville, Tennessee

Lawrence Grunfeld, M.D.
Department of Obstetrics, Gynecology and Reproductive Science, Division of Reproductive Endocrinology, Mount Sinai School of Medicine, New York, New York

Donna M. Kepple, R.T., R.D.M.S.
Department of Radiology and Radiological Sciences, Section of Ultrasound, Vanderbilt University Medical Center, Nashville, Tennessee

Rudy E. Sabbagha, M.D.
Department of Obstetrics and Gynecology, Northwestern University Medical School, Chicago, Illinois

Benjamin Sandler, M.D.
Department of Obstetrics, Gynecology and Reproductive Science, Division of Reproductive Endocrinology, Mount Sinai School of Medicine, New York, New York

Preface

When endovaginal ultrasound arrived in the United States, its initial focus was its obvious application to infertility. Among Ob/Gyns, all subspecialists in reproductive endocrinology and practitioners of in vitro fertilization became aware of this diagnostic modality. Thereafter, its value in early pregnancy, first in earlier recognition of intrauterine gestations, then in the potential for earlier diagnosis of some fetal anomalies, excited many perinatally oriented Ob/Gyns. Above all, now and in the future, endovaginal ultrasound will have the greatest impact in general Ob/Gyn day-to-day practice. This stems from the ability of the modality to be incorporated into the busy routine of such a practice—not merely in the office, not merely as some ancillary procedure in a separate treatment room, but in the examining room itself, for instant clinical correlation in appropriate patients.

For radiologists, endovaginal ultrasound will complement many of the routine pelvic ultrasound studies that are now performed on a daily basis. The cyst that appeared unilocular with a full-bladder transabdominal scan may show fine internal septations on high-frequency endovaginal examination; the markedly enlarged uterus with multiple myomas on transabdominal sector scan may, on endovaginal examination, actually show a separate but adjacent cyst filled with debris—two examples of how endovaginal ultrasound examination can improve diagnostic acumen. Endovaginal ultrasound will also open a host of new sonographically guided procedures: follicle retrieval; diagnostic or therapeutic aspiration of cysts and abscesses; possible conservative treatment of ectopic pregnancy by instillation of substances like methotrexate or potassium chloride; first-trimester prenatal genetic diagnosis; and the controversial situation of selective termination in multiple pregnancies.

Endovaginal ultrasound will play a major role in reshaping the field of imaging. The "laying of hands"—long the credo of the physician—has become somewhat lost to the diagnostic radiologist. Now endovaginal ultrasound will see a joining together of the physical examination and the imaging process. The eliciting of tenderness, if present, has long been a significant aspect of the pelvic exam. Now the ability to examine with an endovaginal probe, the ability to elicit that tenderness while seeing structures in the path of the beam of sound, will cause the diagnostic radiologist to develop expertise in previously unexplored waters. For sonographers, as for Ob/Gyns and radiologists, endovaginal ultrasound is really a specialized form of the pelvic exam.

This text is truly a clinically relevant monograph. Whether you are an Ob/Gyn, a radiologist, or a sonographer, it covers everything you need to know to get started in endovaginal ultrasound. It is my hope that this volume will serve as a basis for beginning to understand and incorporate endovaginal ultrasound as part of your clinical practice.

Steven R. Goldstein, M.D.

Acknowledgments

I have savored, to the very end, this most pleasant task—that of reflecting on all those without whom this book would never have been a reality. Indulge me, however, for this is my first book, and perhaps it is almost like a child. It "gives me pause" (as my wife Kathy would say in her most South Carolinian accent) to sit here and ponder how it came to be.

I want to thank Ira Laufer, M.D., for being that first (and still) special role model; Lewis Shenker, M.D., a mentor figure admired from afar; Riggoberto Santos-Ramos, M.D., for my roots in ultrasound; Dickie Jones, M.D., a very special friend and a wonderful orthopedic surgeon, who helped me understand how to navigate in the waters of academic medicine; Robert F. Porges, M.D., a superb teacher, role model, and now colleague, who always seemed to help me gain entry to the right place at the right time; Bala Subramanyam, M.D., who taught me so much ultrasound and is the best sonographer I know (and I know a lot of sonographers!); George Otey, Roberta Hertig, Peter Becker, Lee Oppegaard, and Carol Bennett, for having faith in a "new kid on the block"; Carol Watson, Eileen Weinstein, Ginny Elwell, and Linda Horwath, for scanning just one more patient; Juanita Castro, for being my third hand in the office; Dr. Milton Danon and everyone at Parkmed Clinic, for enabling me to learn so much about early pregnancy; Kathy Reed, M.D., and Robert Wolfson, M.D., Ph.D., for being the kind of professional acquaintances that evolve into lasting friendships; everyone at Alan R. Liss, Inc., for nurturing the seed within me that was meant to accomplish this goal; Ellen Bloom, for putting up with my handwriting, my endless drafts, and me; Jon Snyder, M.D., for being a very special colleague, friend, and buffer PRN; Howard S. Goldstein, M.D., for being the best big brother a person could ever hope for; Margery Goldstein, my mother, for teaching me to "play fair and square and Even-Steven"; and most of all my wife Kathy Dillon Goldstein, for giving me the peace of mind to settle down, accomplish my goals, and still "smell the roses."

It is a wonderful, warm feeling, and I thank all of you.

Steven R. Goldstein, M.D.
New York City 1988

Why Endovaginal Ultrasound?

Endovaginal ultrasound has the potential to affect the way we practice medicine on many different levels. Initially, even the developers of the new technology saw it as a specialized extension of current imaging techniques and practice patterns. The more one uses and explores endovaginal ultrasound, the more one sees that certain of its applications will be far more advantageous than previously available techniques. However, in other areas not only will it offer no advantage, it will not even approach the level of information now provided.

It will be used in every laboratory or office performing obstetrical and gynecological ultrasound. In addition, however, it will bring scores of physicians previously involved in reproductive endocrinology and infertility into the imaging domain. It will change our concepts of early pregnancy failure. It will either confirm or rewrite the textbooks on embryology in the first trimester of pregnancy, thus allowing for a new wave of first-trimester diagnoses. It will reduce further the gap between the ability to diagnose pregnancy from biochemical signs and to first visualize the embryo within the uterine cavity. Thus it will also enhance our ability to diagnose ectopic pregnancy; it will complement many of our traditional transabdominal ultrasound studies; it will open new horizons in imaging the cervix, the endometrium, and the ovary; it will allow a whole new set of possibilities for ultrasonically guided procedures through the vagina (follicle retrieval, cyst puncture, selective termination, methotrexate, or potassium chloride infusion into ectopics). The technique also offers promise as a potential screening tool in the postmenopausal state looking for malignant disease. Perhaps most important, however, it will find its way into every gynecologic examining room. Although I do not believe it will become as integral a part of the pelvic exam as the speculum, it will perhaps be more on the order of magnitude of a colposcope, being employed in a multitude of situations where it will enhance the clinical exam and offer instant objective documentation of clinical impressions. Of course this raises some ethical issues of intellectual honesty and the conflict of self referral, but the challenge to avoid abuse of this new modality should not hold back the valuable contribution that it has the potential to make.

The cornerstone of its utility is 1) an empty urinary bladder and 2) the clear resolution of the higher frequency tranducers in the near field.

Transabdominal ultrasound traditionally stresses the importance of a filled urinary bladder. The filled urinary bladder effectively displaces gas-filled loops of bowel in a cephalad direction. Bowel filled with liquid and air and the complex echoes this produces has long been one of the bugaboos of ultrasound. This is true of endovaginal scanning as well. How to recognize bowel and not let it interfere with endovaginal scanning is an important element of mastering the technique. The filled urinary bladder acts as an image enhancer often referred to as an "acoustic window." This enhancement is not available in endovaginal scanning, but the lack is compensated for by the increased resolution of the higher frequency transducers used.

The empty urinary bladder will save time and be better tolerated by the patient. It allows for performance of endovaginal ultrasound at the same time as the pelvic exam is performed in the gynecologist's office. The visual record of the ultrasound study can give instant correlation to the subjective findings of traditional bimanual examination.

The other advantage of endovaginal ultrasound—higher frequency allowing superb resolution even with magnification in the near field—is also the basis for its biggest limitation—a very limited field of vision. A slightly enlarged fibroid uterus may not fit in one entire field of vision, yet a 3 cm ovarian cyst fills much of the entire field, making its large sonolucency virtually impossible to overlook, even by the beginner with little or no previous training.

The orientation of the images does take a certain amount of adjustment because the concepts "longitudinal" and "transverse" lose their meaning in endovaginal scanning. This technique uses "anatomy-derived orientation," in which recognizable anatomic structures provide the necessary reference points. Success in endovaginal scanning comes with experience and learning various tricks for finding the anatomical structures in which we are interested.

Perhaps most significant, however, is the introduction of a modality that blurs the boundary between palpation (i.e., the pelvic exam) and imaging: the ability to see structures in the path of the transducer and to incorporate the physical findings (the presence or absence of tenderness) with the images produced; the ability to use an abdominal hand to guide structures to the endovaginal probe. This modality will result more and more in radiologists practicing the art of pelvic physical exam and in obstetricians/gynecologists incorporating imaging into the physical diagnosis portion of their synthesis of the clinical picture.

Chapter 1

How to Begin: Basic Instrumentation and Method of Examination

Endosonography is based upon imaging specific organs with ultrasonic probes placed into adjacent body cavities. For example, the pelvis or the prostate gland can be imaged by endovaginal or endorectal probes. Specific cardiac planes can also be imaged with esophageal probes. Additionally, the peritoneal and uterine cavities can be examined by small probes adapted for use in conjunction with laparoscopy and hysteroscopy. However, the latter techniques are still experimental, and their role in endosonography is not yet defined.

This chapter is limited to endovaginal sonography and includes a discussion of:

1. Basic physics, particularly in relation to the enhanced resolution observed with endosonography.
2. Advantages and limitations of the endovaginal approach.
3. Instrumentation.
4. Method of examination, encompassing physician/patient interaction, necessary preparation, orientation of the scan, and technique of imaging the uterus and adnexae.

This chapter was prepared by Rudy E. Sabbagha, M.D.

PHYSICS

The principles of physics governing the use of vaginal transducers are similar to those applied for external probes. A piezoelectric element or crystal is used to transmit ultrasonic sound waves. The echoes produced from multiple interfaces (areas situated between tissues of varying density) are also received by the same element and subsequently transformed into electric impulses suitable for viewing on a television monitor. The size and shape of the transducer controls the frequency of the emitted ultrasonic waves as well as the length of the near and far fields (Fig. 1–1). The frequency of ultrasound is expressed in Mega-Hertz (MHz) or million vibrations per second. For example, a 2 MHz transducer emits 2 million vibrations per second.

FREQUENCY

It is important that sonographers understand the relationship between ultrasound frequency, wavelength, and velocity. Frequency is related to both velocity and wavelength according to the equation:

$$\text{frequency} = \frac{\text{velocity}}{\text{wavelength}}$$

The velocity of ultrasound varies according to the density of the medium traversed. However, a speed of 1,540 m/sec is accepted as the average velocity in tissues.

Since velocity is a constant, transducers emitting pulses of high-frequency ultrasound, in the range of 5–7 MHz, generate waves of shorter length than those with lower frequencies, in the range of 2–3 MHz. For example, a 7-MHz transducer emits 0.22-mm waves, whereas a 2-MHz transducer emits 0.77-mm waves.

RESOLUTION

Resolution is a term used to define the ability of an ultrasonic machine to individually depict two interfaces situated in close proximity to each other, either axially (along the path of the beam) or laterally (along an axis perpendicular to the beam). Short pulses

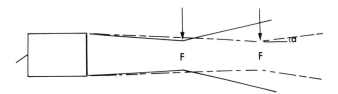

Fig. 1-1. The transducer is shown emitting high-frequency ultrasound (dotted line) and low-frequency ultrasound (solid line). Both near fields end at the points shown by the arrows. The ultrasonic beams in the near fields converge to the focal point (F). Note that with high-frequency ultrasound the length of the near field is long and the beam diameter small. Similarly, with high-frequency ultrasound the angle of divergence (a) in the far field is smaller than that with low-frequency ultrasound.

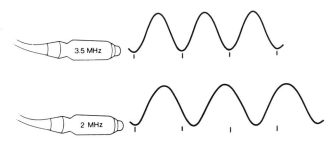

Fig. 1-2. Note that the wavelength emitted by higher-frequency ultrasound (3.5 MHz vs 2 MHz) is small and captures interfaces situated in close proximity to each other.

of high-frequency ultrasound (5–7 MHz) have the capability of resolving interfaces situated within 1.5–1 mm of each other (Fig. 1–2).

Interfaces situated perpendicular to the path of sound waves are also better resolved by higher-frequency waves, because the ultrasonic beam is narrower, the near field is longer, and the angle of divergence in the far field is smaller (Fig. 1–1).

ATTENUATION

Unfortunately, with higher frequency, penetration of ultrasound in tissues is reduced, a phenomenon related to its increased absorption by conversion to heat. Ultrasound can also be attenuated (reflected and refracted) by subcutaneous tissue, as in abdominal sonography, or by bowel, as in endovaginal sonography. However, the recent introduction of *dynamic frequency imaging* has solved at least part of the difficulty attributed to attenuation. With this approach, the transducer transmits a wide variety of frequencies, automatically optimizing the scan frequency in relation to depth.

FOCUSED PROBES

Focusing is achieved by adding an acoustic lens to the surface of the crystal or by the construction of a curved element. The area of focus is defined as that falling within the confines of the narrowest portions of the beam within the near field (Fig. 1–1). Lateral resolution is mainly dependent on the width or diameter of the ultrasonic beam. Beam diameter is narrowed not only by high-frequency ultrasound but also by the use of focused transducers. Additionally, focusing lengthens the near field and decreases the angle of divergence in the far field, thus improving overall resolution (Fig. 1–1).

The length of the near field is also related to the diameter of the transducer, according to the formula:

$$\text{near field} = \frac{(\text{radius of transducer})^2}{\text{wavelength}}$$

For example, the near field of a 2-MHz transducer with a radius of 10 mm is:

Step 1. $(10)^2$/wavelength or 100/wavelength.
Step 2. Since wavelength = velocity/frequency, or
    1,540,000 (mm/sec)/2 $\times$ 10^6, or 0.77 mm,
Step 3. The near field = 100/0.77 mm, or 129.8 mm (12.9 cm).

By contrast, the near field of a 5-MHz transducer with the same crystal is much longer, or 100/0.308 mm or 324.6 mm (32.5 cm).

Real-time dynamic focusing, a technique recently introduced, has further enhanced acoustic focusing. In this technology an electronically shaped acoustic lens, controlled by computer, is focused up to 16 times for each image, keeping the entire field of view in focus.

ENDOVAGINAL APPLICATIONS

The advantage of endovaginal imaging is related to the fact that the probe can be placed in close proximity to pelvic structures. As a result, attenuation is reduced to a minimum, and the pelvic area remains within the focal length of the transducer. The latter two factors permit use of higher-frequency transducers, which in turn markedly enhance the quality of ultrasonic images.

However, there are some limiting factors to endovaginal ultrasound. First, large ovarian or uterine masses extending well into the abdomen cannot be imaged in totality because they are positioned beyond the focal zone of the transducer. Second, a full bladder, considered of great advantage in abdominal imaging, cannot be utilized as a sonic window because its large size will also displace pelvic structures away from the vaginal fornices. Finally, the presence of bowel in the cul-de-sac and adnexal region interferes with the transmission of sound to these areas. Nevertheless, identification of the internal iliac vessels or ovarian follicles will frequently assist the sonographer in localizing the ovaries.

It is important that bowel will not interfere with imaging the uterus and its contents. Thus endovaginal sonography has added a significant dimension in the evaluation of the uterus, particularly during the first trimester of pregnancy.

INSTRUMENTATION

Although real-time linear array transducers have been used endovaginally, sector probes are preferable because they allow superior orientation and localization of pathology within the pelvis.

In the United States the impetus for the development of endovaginal sonography has been the aspiration of ovarian follicles to separate oocytes for in vitro fertilization. For this reason most of the endovaginal transducers in the United States are manufactured to emit a forward-looking sector, varying from 60–110° (Fig. 1–3), an angle that is certainly satisfactory for follicle imaging. Additionally, the majority of the transducers are manufactured with a built-in angulation of the handle (Fig. 1–4), which permits the sonographer to direct and hold the tip of the probe easily in either vaginal fornix.

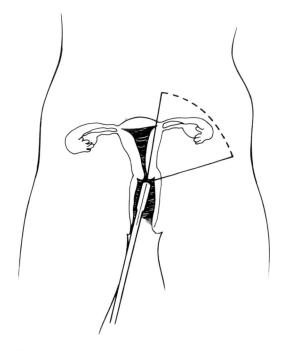

Fig. 1-3. The endovaginal transducer is in the left oblique position, imaging the left adnexa via a forward sector angle of approximately 60°.

In Europe, however, a variety of wide-angled sector probes (> 270°) and 360° rotator scanners have been used. These probes can produce panoramic transverse, sagittal, and coronal views of the pelvis, depending on their orientation in the vaginal canal. They have been successfully used not only for depicting pelvic pathology but also for assessing pelvic size (true conjugate of inlet and interspinous diameter of midpelvis) in women at high risk for dystocia. Some of these probes have also been encased within small water-filled balloons and used to enhance detection of tumor spread in patients with cervical or uterine cancer.

In addition to real-time dynamic frequency imaging and real-time dynamic focusing, convex array technology has recently been utilized in endovaginal sonography. In this technology, sound beams are transmitted and received at right angles to the transducer surface, resulting in naturally steered sector images of superior quality.

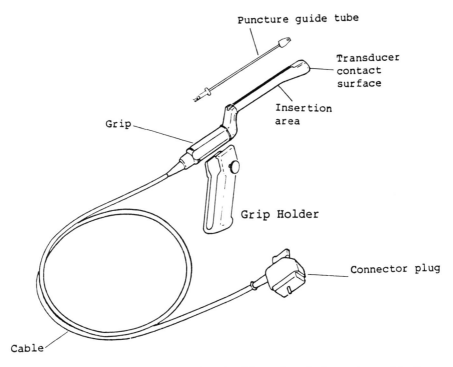

Fig. 1-4. Note the angulation in the handle of the endovaginal transducer; this allows the gynecologist to fix the tip of the transducer comfortably in one of the vaginal fornices for oocyte retrieval from ovarian follicles. Courtesy of Corometrics Medical Systems, Inc.

THE EXAMINATION

Interaction With Patients

It is important that sonographers communicate to patients the importance of endovaginal sonography and assure them that the discomfort, if any, is akin to a regular pelvic examination. Overall, endovaginal sonography has been well accepted by patients. Initially, they react positively to the fact that the examination is conducted with an empty or near empty bladder. Subsequently, they feel enthused about the crispness of the image and their ability to participate in its interpretation, particularly when it comes to counting follicles or observing the early small fetus with its beating heart.

Preparation

The transducer should be covered by a condom filled with approximately 5 ml of ultrasonic gel. Surgilube is then applied to the examiner's glove and used to lubricate the walls of the vagina.

When the uterus is markedly anteverted, the examination can be conducted in one of three ways. In the first way the patient is placed in lithotomy position, allowing the examiner to freely angle the tip of the transducer upward, in the direction of the uterus (Fig. 1-5). This maneuver may not be possible if the patient is in supine position because motion of the transducer handle downward (to achieve elevation of its tip) will be limited by the examination table. Alternatively, placement of a folded pillow or a 4–6-inch foam pad under the pelvis will produce enough elevation to allow downward movement of the transducer handle.

Finally, it is possible to rotate the transducer 180° so that the angulation of the handle is pointing upward toward the symphysis pubis. This will allow the operator to direct the tip of the transducer anteriorly. Furthermore, in the transverse plane the orientation is such that the right side of the patient now appears on the right side of the image and vice versa.

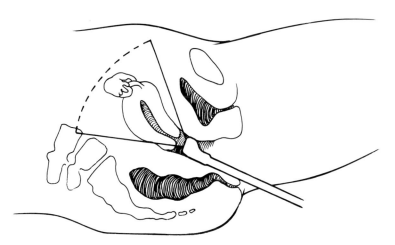

Fig. 1-5. Note the upward angulation of the tip of the transducer necessary for visualization of an anteverted uterus. To achieve this angle, the sonographer must direct the handle toward the table, a procedure that may not be possible unless the patient is in lithotomy position, or the pelvis elevated by using a 4-6 inch pad, or the transducer handle rotated 180° (see text). If the uterus is retroverted, the transducer handle should be held upward, i.e., in the opposite direction.

Orientation

Once the preparation is complete, the sonographer gently inserts the transducer into the vagina with the marker pointing anteriorly toward the symphysis pubis. Its handle is then moved downward, toward the table (Fig. 1–5). This maneuver will produce a sagittal image of the uterus. At this point the orientation of the image in relation to the bladder should be checked. Even though the bladder is nearly empty, its walls can still be readily identified. Unlike abdominal sonography, the bladder should appear on the left side of the screen. However, this is not universally agreed upon, and some sonographers still place it on the right.

The extent to which a uterus is anteverted or retroverted determines 1) the depth of transducer insertion; and 2) optimal angulation in relation to the vaginal axis. Maneuvering the transducer by withdrawal and reinsertion at different angles will allow the operator to locate and capture the best image of the uterus and its contents. The sonographer should then proceed to evaluate the uterus transversely. This is done by rotating the transducer so that the marker is facing the right upper thigh. In this way the right aspect of the patient's uterus will appear on the left side of the screen and vice versa (Fig. 1–6).

Determining the orientation of the uterus in the transverse plane may be of importance in assessing clinical scenarios associated with congenital anomalies of the uterus, for example, bicornuate uterus (Fig. 1–6). Additionally, the correct orientation may be important in evaluating the location of a myoma as well as its size and its proximity to the endometrial cavity. Such information may assist the gynecologist in determining whether an indicated myomectomy should be performed by means of operative hysteroscopy or laparotomy.

Having completed the examination of the uterus, the transducer marker is rotated to an oblique position. In this way the tip of the transducer will be facing the right adnexa. At this point bowel is encountered, making localization of the normal right ovary somewhat difficult. Nonetheless, with experience the sonographer will be able to see the boundaries of the ovary adjacent to the internal iliac vessels. Even though the right adnexa is being examined, the image of the right ovary will occupy the central portion of the screen (Fig. 1–7). Thus it is important for the sonographer to keep in mind the oblique direction of the probe and to adequately label the echogram (Fig. 1–8). For example,

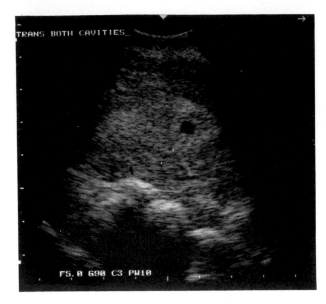

Fig. 1–6. Transverse scan of a bicornuate uterus produced by an endovaginal probe with marker rotated to the patient's right thigh. In the sagittal plane the bladder was on the right side of the screen. The right uterine horn is seen on the left side of the image and shows a decidual reaction. The left uterine horn is seen on the right side of the image and shows an early intrauterine pregnancy.

the label should indicate that the photograph represents an endovaginal examination of the ovary in the right oblique orientation. A similar method of examination is used for the left adnexa, and the photograph is labeled accordingly (Fig. 1–3).

Despite our inability to measure the size of large adnexal masses, endovaginal imaging of ovarian tumors has yielded valuable preoperative information. The benefit over abdominal scans has been in the more accurate delineation of internal echo characteristics. Specifically, some ovarian tumors that appeared totally cystic when imaged abdominally have shown a variety of internal echo patterns with endovaginal probes. For example, in many patients, septations, diffusely homogeneous fine echoes (as with endometriosis), and even papillary projections have only been apparent with vaginal probes.

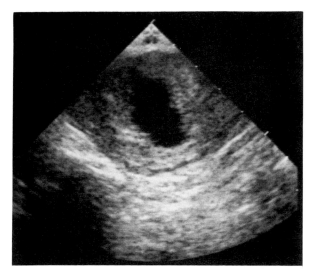

Fig. 1–7. Sonogram obtained by endovaginal transducer facing the right adnexa and placed in the right oblique position. However, the image of the right ovary displaying a cyst (consistent with corpus luteum cyst) is seen in the middle of the screen. Appropriate labeling of the scan is necessary (see text).

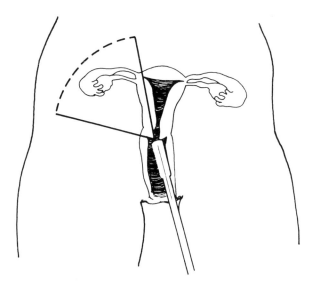

Fig. 1–8. Demonstration of the right oblique position of the endovaginal transducer used to produce the image in Figure 1-7.

SUGGESTED READINGS

Bernaschek G. Endosonography. In Sabbagha RE (ed): Diagnostic Ultrasound Applied to Obstetrics and Gynecology, Ed 2. Philadelphia: J.B. Lippincott, 1987, Chapter 44.

Bernaschek G, Deutinger J, Bart W, Janisch H. Endosonographic staging of carcinoma of the uterine cervix. Arch Gynecol 239:21, 1986.

Campbell S, Goessens L, Goswany R, et al. Real-time ultrasonography for determination of ovarian morphology and volume. A possible early screening test for ovarian cancer. Lancet 1:425, 1982.

Dellenbach P, Nisand I, Moreau L, et al. Transvaginal sonographically controlled follicle puncture for oocyte retrieval. Fertil Steril 44:656, 1985.

Deutinger J, Bernaschek G. Die vaginal sonographische pelvimetrie als weur methode zur sonographischen Bestimmung der inneren Beckenmabe. Geburtshilfe Frauenheilkd 46:345, 1986.

Granberg S, Wikland M. Comparison between endovaginal and transabdominal transducers for measuring ovarian volume. J Ultrasound Med 6:649, 1987.

Lenz S, Lauritsen JG, Kjellow M. Collection of human oocytes for in vitro fertilization by ultrasonically guided follicular puncture. Lancet 1:1163, 1981.

Popp LW, Lueken RP, Lindemann HJ. Hysterosonographie. Diagn Intersither 4:69, 1982.

Schwimer SR, Lebovic J. Transvaginal pelvic ultrasonography. J Ultrasound Med 4:61, 1985.

Timor-Tritsch IE, Rottem S., Thaler I. Review of transvaginal ultrasonography: A description with clinical applications. Ultrasound 6:1, 1988.

Vilaro MM, Rifkin MD, Pennell RG, et al. Endovaginal ultrasound: A technique for evaluation of nonfollicular pelvic masses. J Ultrasound Med 6:697, 1987.

Watanabe H, Saitoh M, Mishina T, et al. Mass screening program for prostatic diseases with transrectal ultrasonography. J Urol 117:746–748, 1977.

Chapter 2

Normal Pelvic Anatomy: What You Can Expect to See

Endovaginal sonography gives better resolution of the uterus and ovaries than does the conventional transabdominal approach. While the proximity of the transducer/probe to the pelvic organs allows their more detailed depiction, it may be more, rather than less, difficult for the sonographer to become oriented to the images obtained on an endovaginal sonogram, compared with conventional, transabdominal sonography, since endovaginal sonography has a limited field of view and unusual scanning planes. However, as one develops a systematic approach to the examination of the uterus and adnexal structures with endovaginal sonography, the examination becomes easier. In this chapter, the sonographic appearances of the uterus, ovary, and other adnexal and pelvic structures will be described, with particular emphasis on how they are best depicted upon real-time, endovaginal sonographic examination.

SCANNING TECHNIQUE AND INSTRUMENTATION

The three scanning maneuvers that are used in endovaginal ultrasound include.

1. Vaginal insertion of the probe, with side-to-side movement within the upper vagina for sagittal imaging.

This chapter was prepared by Arthur C. Fleischer, M.D., and Donna M. Kepple, R.T., R.D.M.S.

2. Transverse orientation of the probe for imaging in various degrees of semiaxial-to-axial planes.
3. Variation in probe insertion for optimal imaging of the fundus to cervix by gradual withdrawal of the probe into the lower vagina for cervical imaging.

As opposed to conventional transabdominal ultrasound, bladder distension is not required for the endovaginal exam. In fact, overdistension can hinder the exam by placing the desired field of view outside the optimal focal range of the transducer. Minimal distension is useful in a patient with a severely anteflexed uterus to straigthen it out relative to the imaging plane.

As is true for conventional sonographic equipment, one should select the highest frequency transducer possible that allows adequate penetration and depiction of a particular region of interest. Thus 5- to 7.5-MHz transducers are preferred, but these higher-frequency transducers limit the field-of-view to only within 6 cm of the probe.

The major types of transducer/probes utilized for endovaginal scanning include those that contain a single-element oscillating transducer, those with multiple small transducer elements arranged in a curved linear array, and those that consist of multiple small elements steered by an electronic phased array (see Chapter 3). All three types depict the anatomy in a sector format that usually encompasses 100°. In our experience, the greatest resolution is achieved with a curved linear array that contains multiple (up to 124) separate transmit-receive elements. Mechanical sector transducers may be subject to major image distortions at the edges of the field because of the hysteresis (stopping and starting) that occurs with an oscillating transducer. Although degradation of image quality by side lobe artifacts can occur in the far field in a phased array transducer, they do not significantly degrade the image in the near field. Therefore phased array transducers have resolution capabilities similar to sector and curved linear transducers for use in endovaginal examinations.

After complete covering of the transducer/probe by a condom, sheath, or finger of a rubber glove, the probe is inserted within the vagina and manipulated around the cervical lips and into the fornix so as to depict the structures of interest in best detail. When the transducer is oriented in the longitudinal or sagittal plane, the long axis of the uterus can usually be depicted by slight angulation off midline. The uterus is used as a landmark for depiction of other adnexal structures. Once the uterus is identified, the probe can be angled to the right or left of midline in the sagittal plane to depict the ovaries. The internal iliac artery and vein appear as tubular structures along the pelvic sidewall. Low-level blood echoes can occasionally be seen streaming within these pulsating vessels. The ovaries typically lie medial to them. After appropriate images are obtained in the sagittal plane, the transducer can be turned 90° to depict these structures in their axial or semicoronal planes.

Particularly in larger patients, it is helpful for the sonographer to use one hand to scan while the other is used for gentle abdominal palpation, so as to move structures such as the ovaries as close as possible to the transducer/probe.

UTERUS

Examination of the uterus begins with its depiction in long axis. The endometrial interface, which is typically echogenic, is a useful landmark to depict the long axis of the uterus. Once the endometrium is identified, images of the uterus can be obtained in the sagittal and semiaxial/coronal plane (Fig. 2–1).

It may be difficult to determine the flexion of the uterus on the hard copy images obtained from endovaginal scanning alone, except in extreme cases of ante- or retroflexion. However, one can obtain an impression of a uterine flexion during the examination by the relative orientation of the transducer/probe needed to obtain the most optimal images of the uterus. For example, retroflexed uteri are best depicted when the probe is in the anterior fornix and angulated in a posterior direction.

The endometrium has a variety of appearances, depending on its stage of development. In the proliferative phase (Fig. 2–2), the endometrium measures 3–5 mm in anterior-posterior (AP) dimension (width). This measurement includes two layers of endometrium. A hypoechoic interface can be seen within the luminal aspects of echogenic layers of endometrium in the periovulatory phase and probably represents an edema in the inner layers of endometrium. In the few days after ovulation (Fig. 2–3A,B), a small amount of secretion into the endometrial lumen can be seen. During the secretory phase (Fig. 2–4), the endometrium typically measures between 5 and 8 mm in width and is surrounded by a hypoechoic band representing the inner layer of the

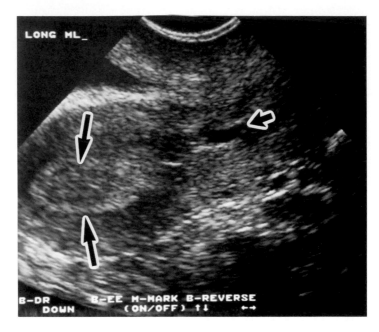

Fig. 2-1. Long axis of uterus in semicoronal plane showing endometrium (large arrows) and cervix. There is a small amount of fluid (small arrow) within the endocervical canal.

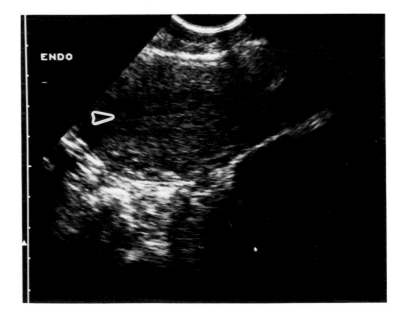

Fig. 2-2. Long axis of endometrium (arrowhead) during the proliferative phase. It is hypoechoic at this stage of development.

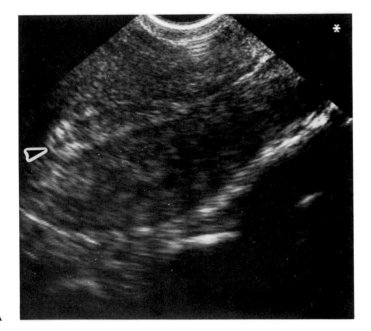

Fig. 2-3. (**A**) Long axis of endometrium (arrowhead) during the periovulatory phase, showing hypoechoic inner layer. (**B**) Same as **A** in short axis. The multilayered endometrium is clearly seen between the +s.

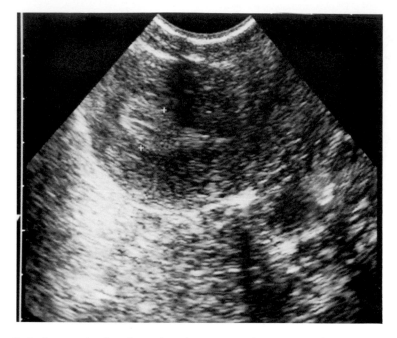

Fig. 2-4. Long axis of endometrium between +s in secretory phase, appearing as echogenic tissue.

myometrium. An endometrial volume may be calculated by measuring its length by long axis, with AP and transverse dimensions. One can use the landmark in the axial plane where the endometrium invaginates into the area of ostia in the region of the uterine cornu.

Because of the proximity of the transducer/probe to the cervix, the cervix is not as readily depicted as the remainder of the uterus. However, if one withdraws the probe into the vagina, images of the cervix can be obtained (Fig. 2-5). The mucus within the endocervical canal usually appears as an echogenic interface. This may become hypoechoic during the periovulatory period, as the cervical mucus has a higher fluid content.

The outer surface of the myometrium will often display small sonolucencies corresponding to the arcuate vessels (Fig. 2-6). Their appearance may vary with different times of the menstrual cycle.

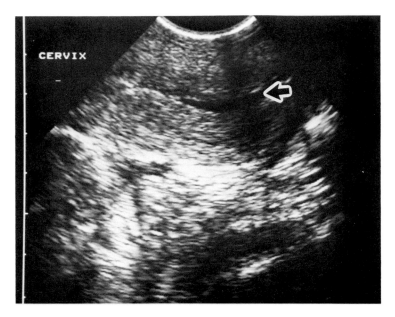

Fig. 2-5. Same patient as in Figure 2-1 after withdrawing the probe into the midvagina. The endocervical canal with its hypoechoic mucus (arrow) is clearly seen.

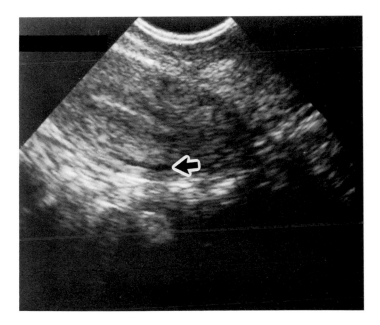

Fig. 2-6. Oblique image showing veins (arrow) within the outer myometrium.

OVARIES

Ovaries are typically depicted as oblong structures measuring approximately 3 cm in long axis and 2 cm in anterior-posterior and transverse dimensions. On angled long axis scans, they are immediately medial to the pelvic vessels. They are particularly well depicted when they contain a mature follicle typically in the 1.5–2.0-cm range (Fig. 2–7). It is not unusual to depict multiple immature or atetric follicles in the 3-mm range.

The size of an ovary is related to the patient's age and phase of follicular development. When the ovary contains a mature follicle, it can become twice as large in volume as one that does not contain mature follicles. A fresh corpus luteum can often be distinguished from a mature follicle by the presence of internal echoes (Fig. 2–8). However, the greatest dimension of a normal ovary typically is less than 3 cm.

OTHER PELVIC STRUCTURES

Endovaginal sonography can depict several other pelvic structures besides the uterus and ovaries. These include bowel loops

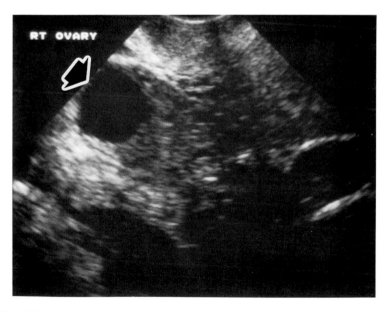

Fig. 2–7. Right ovary containing a mature follicle (arrow) in a spontaneous cycle.

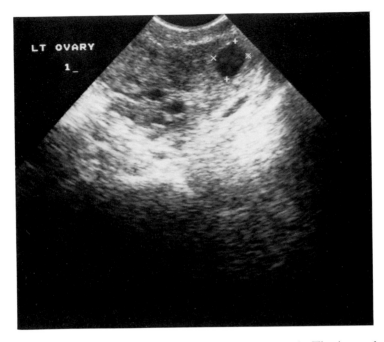

Fig. 2-8. Left ovary containing a fresh corpus luteum (+s). The internal echoes probably arise from clotted blood within the corpus luteum.

within the pelvis, iliac vessels, and occasionally distended Fallopian tubes. Even small amounts (1–3 cc) of intraperitoneal fluid can be detected in the cul-de-sac or surrounding the uterus (Fig. 2–9).

As previously mentioned, the pelvic vessels appear as straight tubular structures on either pelvic side wall (Fig. 2–10). The internal iliac arteries have a typical width of between 5 mm and 7 mm and tend to pulsate with expansion of both walls, whereas the iliac vein is larger (approximately 1 cm) but does not demonstrate this pulsation. Occasionally, low-level "blood echoes" will be seen streaming within the vein. The transducer can be manipulated or pivoted to demonstrate these vessels in their long axis. Occasionally, a distended distal ureter may have this appearance but not demonstrate pulsations. In most patients, the larger branches of the uterine vessels will be demonstrable by endovaginal sonography as tubular structures coursing in the paracervical area.

The nondistended Fallopian tube is difficult to depict on endovaginal sonography, probably because of its small intraluminal size and serpiginous course. Occasionally one can identify the origin of the tubes by finding the invagination of endometrium depicting the area of the tubal ostia and following these structures laterally in the axial or coronal plane. The ovarian and infundibulopelvic ligaments usually cannot be depicted.

Sonographic delineation of the tubes is facilitated by intraperitoneal fluid that may be present in the cul-de-sac. By placing the patient in a reverse Trendelenburg positon, the fluid can be collected around the tube. When surrounded by fluid, the normal tube appears as a 1-cm tubular echogenic structure that usually comes from the lateral aspect of the uterine cornu posterolaterally into the adnexal regions and cul-de-sac (Fig. 2–11). The flaring of the fimbriated end of the tube can be appreciated, in some patients, as it approximates its nearby ovary. Endosonographic depiction of the tube is also facilitated when it contains intraluminal fluid.

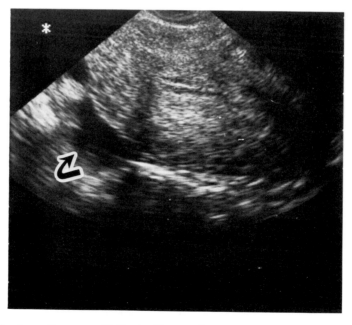

Fig. 2–9. A small amount (3–5 cc) of intraperitoneal fluid (curved arrow) surrounding the uterine fundus, probably secondary to ovulation.

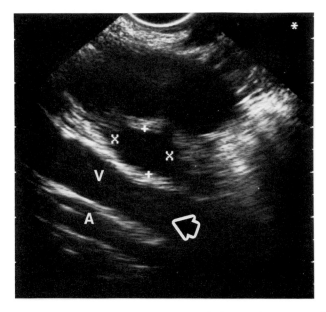

Fig. 2-10. Internal iliac vein (V) and artery (A) in long axis (arrow) adjacent to a follicle-containing ovary.

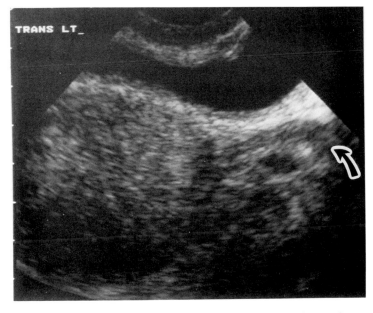

Fig. 2-11. Normal left uterine tube shown in its entire course. Arrow shows portion distal. Uterus is proximal. Small amount of urine in bladder anteriorly appears hypoechoic.

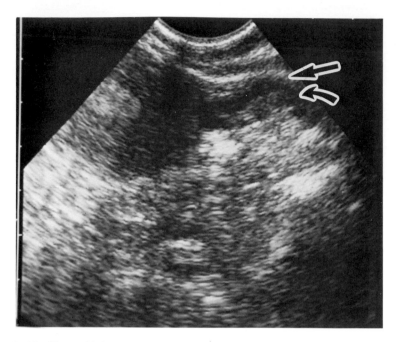

Fig. 2–12. Normal left tube (curved arrow) arising from cornual area adjacent to the uterine attachment of the round ligament (straight arrow).

The endosonographic appearance of the round ligament is somewhat similar to that arising from a nondistended tube, except that its course is more straight and parallel to the uterine cornu (Fig. 2–12).

Bowel can typically be recognized as a fusiform structure that frequently contains intraluminal fluid and changes in configuration because of active peristalsis. If there is fluid within the lumen, periodic intraluminal projections resulting from the valvulae conniventes can be recognized from small bowel (Fig. 2–13A,B), or the haustral indentations that are characteristic of large bowel.

SUMMARY

Endovaginal sonography affords detailed depiction of the uterus and ovaries. However, it requires a systematic evaluation of these pelvic structures for their complete delineation, in light of the limited field of view of endovaginal transducer/probes. This can

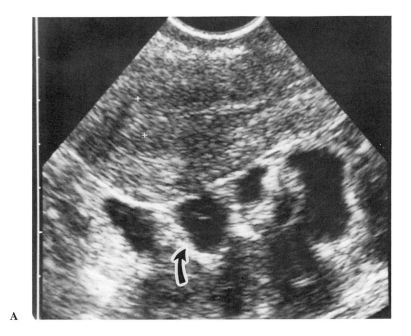

A

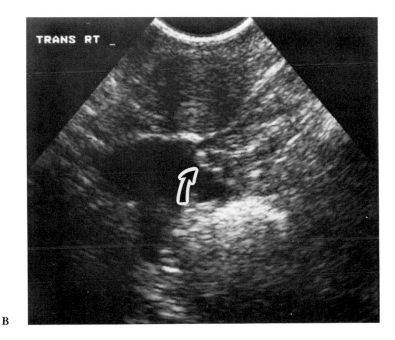

B

Fig. 2-13. (A) Fluid-filled small bowel adjacent to the uterus (curved arrow). **(B)** Contracted small bowel loop (curved arrow) surrounded by intraperitoneal fluid.

be achieved by understanding the anatomical relationship of these structures from prior experience with transabdominal sonography, combined with the anticipated findings from prior palpation of these structures during a pelvic examination.

SUGGESTED READINGS

Fleischer AC, Mendelson E, Bohm-Velez M. Sonographic depiction of the endometrium with transabdominal and transvaginal scanning. Semin Ultrasound CT MRI 9:81–101, 1988.

Granberg S, Wikland M. Comparison between endovaginal and transabdominal transducers for measuring ovarian volume. J Ultrasound Med 16:649–654, 1987.

Timor-Tritsch IE, Rottem S. Transvaginal ultrasonographic study of the Fallopian tube. Obstet Gynecol 70:424–428,1987.

Chapter 3

Pelvic Masses: Endovaginal Sonographic Appearance

Endovaginal sonography has an important role in the evaluation of the uterus and adnexa. However, due to its limited field of view and unusual image orientation, it is best used as an adjunct to a standard transabdominal scan. In particular, endovaginal sonography is indicated for:

1. Determination of the presence or absence and evaluation of relatively small (less than 5–10 cm) adnexal masses.
2. Determination of the origin of a mass (uterine, ovarian, or tubal).
3. Detailed evaluation of its internal consistency, with particular emphasis on the presence or absence of polypoid excrescences, septations, or internal consistencies (blood, pus, serous fluid).
4. Guiding endovaginal aspiration of certain masses.
5. Evaluation of endometrial or myometrial disorders related to pelvic masses.

For masses less than 10 cm in size, endovaginal sonography can afford detailed delineation of the mass and determine its origin. Specifically, masses that arise or are contained within the ovary can be differentiated from those that are intrauterine (Fig. 3–1). Tubal disorders can be identified with this technique, particularly if an abnormally dilated or thickened tube is present (Fig. 3–2).

This chapter was prepared by Arthur C. Fleischer, M.D.

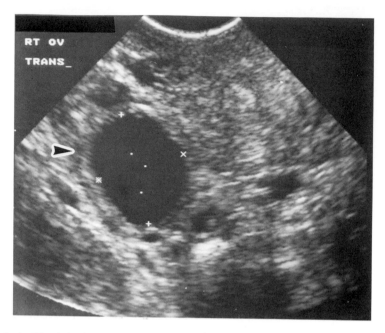

Fig. 3-1. Physiologic cyst (between +s) within right ovary. The compressed ovarian tissue (arrowhead) identifies this mass as being intraovarian.

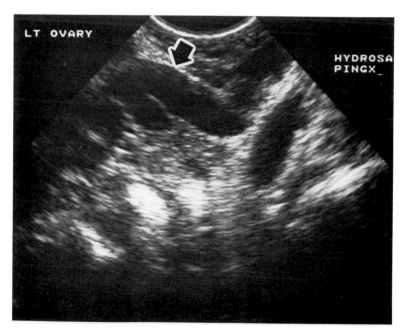

Fig. 3-2. Simple hydrosalpinx (arrow) appearing as fusiform anechoic adnexal structure.

This is particularly helpful in distinguishing inflammatory disorders that may involve the tube and/or ovary, such as a tubo-ovarian abscess (Fig. 3-3) from simple hydrosalpinx. The relative mobility of the pelvic organs can also be assessed when the probe comes into contact with the uterus or ovary.

Endovaginal sonography is particularly helpful in patients with fibroids, since the ovaries can be identified as separate from the uterine abnormality. However, because of high magnification and short focal zone, other myomatous uteri will not entirely fit on the monitor screen. Conversely, some masses that are associated with uterine disorders such as tubo-ovarian abscess with associated endometritis can be identified.

Endovaginal sonography has been used as a means to guide abscess drainage. It is conceivable that simple cysts with serous fluid could be safety aspirated using endovaginal ultrasound. However, "complicated" cysts such as endometriomas, dermoid cysts, or neoplastic cysts have a chance of producing peritonitis or peritoneal spread from rupture and probably should not be aspirated.

Endovaginal sonography affords a means for endovaginal aspiration of those pelvic masses that are thought to be benign serous cysts. Specifically, these masses should demonstrate a smooth and well-defined border with no internal echoes. The sonographer should be aware that low-level artifactural echoes can be observed most with the higher frequency transducer/probes even with some completely serous cysts. The ultrasound findings of calcification, gravity-dependent layering material, or papillary excrescences should dissuade consideration of endovaginal aspiration, since these may indicate "complicated" cysts (Figs. 3-4, 3-5, 3-6). Specifically, there is a chance of iatrogenic production of peritonitis from rupture of an endometrioma or dermoid cyst, of pseudomyxoma peritonei from mucinous tumors, or of peritoneal implants for malignant cystic neoplasms. Regardless of these limitations, however, there may be a role for endovaginal aspiration with or without instillation of sclerosing agents for simple serous cysts. More extensive experience with follow-up after aspiration is needed before the clinical utility and indications for this procedure will be clear.

Although it is tempting to speculate on the use of sonography as a means for screening for ovarian carcinoma in postmenopausal women, the incidence of this disorder requires that hundreds of patients be scanned for a single positive examination. In addition, most masses that are less than 5 cm in size are benign. Clearly,

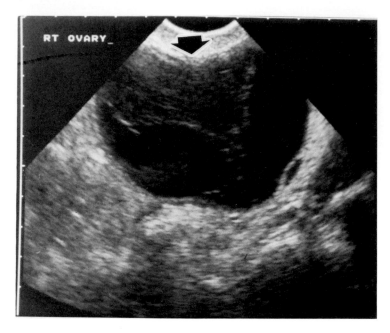

Fig. 3-3. Hemorrhagic corpus luteum cyst appearing as a complex mass. The solid area (arrow) represents compressed ovarian tissue.

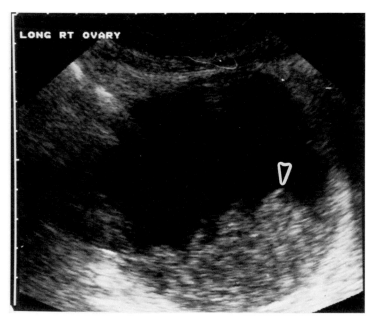

Fig. 3-4. Ovarian tumor with irregular solid contents corresponding to papillary projections (arrowhead).

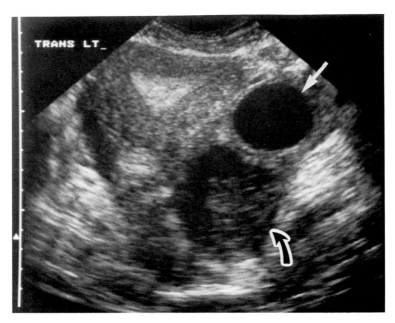

Fig. 3-5. Endometrioma (curved arrow) appearing as a cystic mass containing internal solid materials shown here superior to a mature follicle (straight arrow).

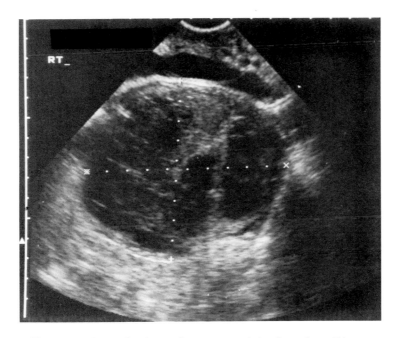

Fig. 3-6. Hemorrhagic ovarian cyst containing irregular solid areas.

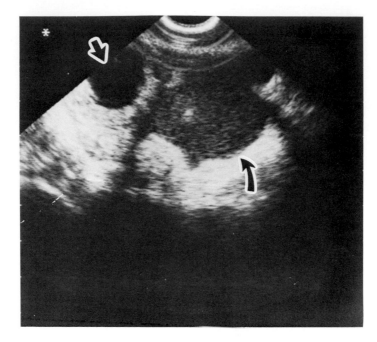

Fig. 3-7. Loculated clotted blood (curved arrow) adjacent to a ruptured corpus luteum cyst (straight arrow). The clotted blood appeared as mildly echogenic semifluid material compared with the contents of the corpus luteum cyst.

however, endovaginal ultrasound has a role in delineation of the ovaries in obese, postmenopausal women in whom the incidence of carcinoma is high and pelvic exam is frequently less than optimal.

Additional investigation is necessary to determine whether the improved resolution afforded by endovaginal sonography of the internal content of a mass would actually aid in its diagnostic specificity. However, our initial impressions, based on 3 years of experience, is that endovaginal ultrasound adds diagnostically specific information in over three-fourths of women studied. Endovaginal ultrasound is particularly helpful in determining the origin of a pelvic mass (intra- or extraovarian) and in documenting tubal, endometrial, and myometrial disorders. The endovaginal approach adds sensitivity over the transabdominal approach, particularly in obese patients.

On endovaginal ultrasound, masses that may appear hypoechoic on transabdominal sonography frequently demonstrate echogenic material suspended within the mass. The echogenic material most frequently represents blood in various degrees of coagulation (Fig. 3–7). However, pus, mucus, or sebaceous material may be echogenic. Thus it may be difficult to distinguish hemorrhagic from neoplastic cysts with endovaginal ultrasound.

In summary, the major roles of endovaginal sonography for evaluation of adnexal masses include demonstration of origin and internal consistency as well as a means for guided aspiration. Endovaginal aspiration may have a role in guidance for aspiration of those masses that appear to be benign by clinical and sonographic criteria. Specifically, because of the remote possibility of peritoneal spillage after an aspiration procedure, one should limit the application of endovaginal aspiration to those masses that appear to be completely cystic, with well-defined borders within freely mobile adnexal structures.

SUGGESTED READINGS

Campbell S, Gosany R. Screening for ovarian carcinoma with ultrasound. Clin Obstet Gynecol 10:621–643, 1984.

Fleischer A, Entman S, Gordon A. Transvaginal sonography of pelvic masses: Does it add specificity? Obstet Gynecol (in press), 1988.

Goldstein SR, Subramanyam BR, Snyder JR, et al. The postmenopausal cystic adnexal mass: The potential role of ultrasound in conservative management. Presented at the Annual Clinical Meeting, American College of Obstetricians and Gynecologists, Boston, Massachusetts, 1988.

Lande IM, Hill MC, Cosco FE, Kator NN. Adnexal and cul-de-sac abnormalities: Transvaginal sonography. Radiology 166:325–332, 1988.

Mendelson EB, Bohm-Velez M, Joseph N, et al. Gynecologic imaging: Comparison of transabdominal and transvaginal sonography. Radiology 166:321–324, 1988.

Nosher JL, Winchman HK, Needell GS. Transvaginal pelvic abscess drainage with US guidance. Radiology 165:872–873, 1987.

Rulin MC, Preston AL. Adnexal masses in postmenopausal women. Obstet Gynecol 70:578–581, 1987.

Timor-Tritsch I, Rottem S (eds). Transvaginal Sonography. New York: Elsevier, 1988, pp 125–141.

Vilaro MM, Rifkin MD, Pennell RG, et al. Endovaginal ultrasound: A technique for evaluation of nonfollicular pelvic masses. J Ultrasound Med 6:697–701, 1987.

Chapter 4

Pregnancy I: Embryo

The first trimester of pregnancy forms a special bridge between the fields of obstetrics and gynecology. Even those who consider themselves specialists limited to either obstetrics or gynecology frequently come in close contact with patients who are clinically in the first trimester.

This book is primarily a text of ultrasound and, more particularly, endovaginal ultrasound. This chapter and the ones that follow aim to show the reader normal and abnormal situations of pregnancy one might encounter clinically, to present the sonographic appearance of such situations, to explain why they appear as they do, and to give some context into which one can incorporate the images into overall clinical practice.

SONOGRAPHIC ASPECTS OF EMBRYOLOGICAL BEGINNINGS

The physiology and anatomy of fertilization and implantation is not sonographically relevant, as unfortunately it is beyond the scope and capabilities of our current equipment. The earliest sonographic changes associated with pregnancy are extremely subtle. Almost from conception the hormonal changes of pregnancy result in increased blood flow for the still undeveloped gestation. Such an increase results in a thickening of the already echogenic postovulatory endometrium, as well as an increase in the prominence of the arcuate vessels in the myometrium (Fig. 4–1). These subtle findings are not diagnostic of pregnancy in and of themselves. The first reliable indicator of an intrauterine ges-

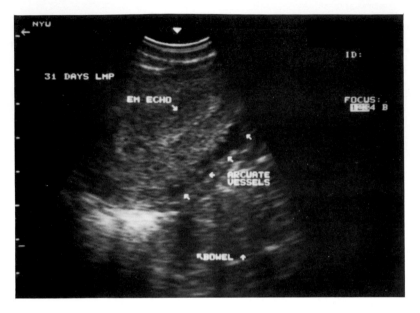

Fig. 4–1. Endovaginal scan at 31 days last menstrual period (LMP). Note the prominent endometrial echo. Arcuate vessels have become quite prominent (multiple small arrows). These changes are subtle and are not definitively diagnostic of pregnancy.

tation is the development of the "gestational sac" (an ultrasound term) (Fig. 4–2).

GESTATIONAL SAC

The blastocyst implants by burrowing into the decidualized endometrium. Already the blastocyst consists of a small amniotic cavity, a bilaminar embryonic disc, and the primary yolk sac (Fig. 4–3). Proliferation of trophoblast produces clumps that form the primary chorionic villi (Fig. 4–4). The early gestational sac is the visualization of an echogenic rind around a sonolucent center (Fig. 4–5). The sonolucent center is the chorionic cavity. It already contains the embryonic disc, amnion, and yolk sac, but they are not well developed and are too small to see even with the high-resolution, highly magnified endovaginal probes currently in use. The echogenic rind is from the trophoblastic decidual reac-

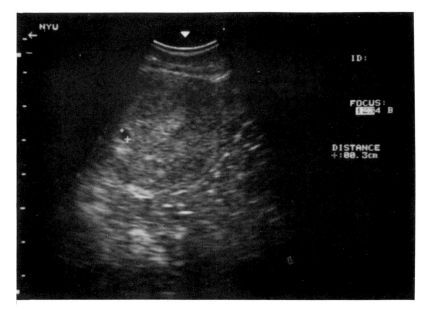

Fig. 4-2. Definitive intrauterine gestational sac (3 mm). Patient has uncertain menstrual history. Beta hCG level was 1,280 mIU/ml (IRP).

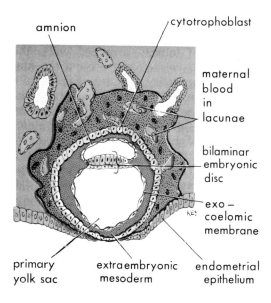

Fig. 4-3. Drawing of a blastocyst approximately 9 days postconception implanted in the endometrium. Note the relationship of the primary yolk sac, the bilaminar embryonic disc, and the amnion. Although all of these structures exist at this early stage, we are not yet able to image them with endovaginal ultrasound techniques. (Reproduced with permission from Keith L. Moore, *The Developing Human*, 4th ed. Philadelphia, W.B. Saunders Co., 1988.)

tion, a result of the invasion of the primary villi (fetal origin) into maternal decidua. Eventually part of these villi will progress, bud, and branch into secondary and tertiary villous projections, and become known as chorion frondosum, which is the forerunner of the placenta. The remaining primary chorionic villi will regress and become known as chorion laeve. At this primary villous stage, the projections are quite symmetrical, regular, and round. Their shaggy appearance accounts for the sonographic image described above (Fig. 4-6). This gestational sac will occasionally be seen before the two layers of decidua fuse. The decidua under the

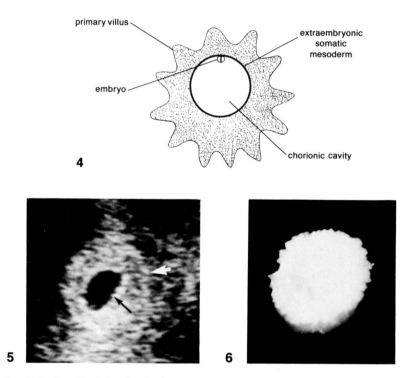

Fig. 4-4. Detail of the chorionic sac. This illustrates the primary villi as they begin to invade the maternal decidua. Note the presence but relative size of the embryo (see Fig. 4-3) at this stage.

Fig. 4-5. Endovaginal scan of 9-mm gestational sac. The echogenic rind (large arrow) is the result of trophoblastic decidual reaction. The sonolucent center (small arrow) represents the chorionic cavity.

Fig. 4-6. Pathology specimen at 5.5 weeks LMP. Note the chorionic cavity with primary villi projecting throughout. This creates the shaggy appearance, which results in the echogenic rind as these villi invade maternal decidua.

blastocyst is decidua basalis. The decidua overlying the embryo is decidua capsularis. The remainder of the endometrial cavity is lined by decidua parietalis. As the gestation grows, the decidua capsularis and parietalis will fuse. Occasionally one will see the remaining endometrial cavity with a central sonolucency adjacent to the eccentric gestational sac. This probably represents a small amount of blood from implantation bleeding (Fig. 4–7A,B).

EARLY PREGNANCY DETECTION

One of the most valuable future applications of endovaginal ultrasound will be its enhanced ability to diagnose pregnancy earlier than traditional transabdominal ultrasound techniques. Biochemically we can diagnose pregnancy by serum radioimmune assay as early as 10 days postconception. Previously there was as much as a 4-week window between the time of biochemical diagnosis and the time when an intrauterine gestation (IUG) could be imaged reliably and definitively. Thus the concept of a "discriminatory zone" of human chorionic gonadotropin (hCG) was first

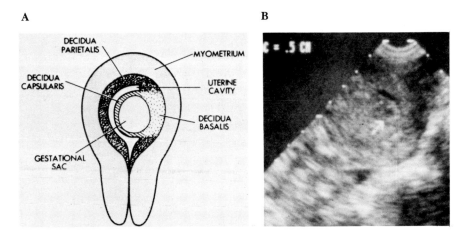

A **B**

Fig. 4–7. (A) Line drawing showing eccentric implantation of gestation under decidua capsularis. Note decidua capsularis and decidua parietalis not yet fused. **(B)** Endovaginal ultrasound revealing eccentrically located gestational sac of 5 mm maximal sac diameter. Adjacent sonolucency probably represents some implantation bleeding between decidua capsularis and decidua parietalis.

introduced. This is the level of hCG above which normal intra-uterine pregnancies should virtually all be imaged within the uterine cavity. Obviously, extrauterine or abnormal intrauterine pregnancies might not be imaged within the uterus in spite of hCG levels greater than this discriminatory zone.

Standards for Measurement of hCG Levels (mIU/ml)
International Reference Preparation (IRP)
Second International Standard (2nd IS)

At this point the reader must be aware that there are two standards for reporting milli-international units (mIU) of hCG. An original discriminatory zone of 6,000–6,500 mIU/ml was reported in the International Reference Preparation (IRP). A modification of the discriminatory zone to 1,800 mIU/ml was actually standardized according to the Second International Standard (2nd IS). The 2nd IS values are approximately one-half the IRP values. Therefore, the more recent "discriminatory zone" is actually at the level of 3,600 mIU/ml (IRP).

All previous work on trying to define a "discriminatory zone" of hCG was done with traditional transabdominal ultrasound scanning techniques. Higher frequency endovaginal probes have allowed us to image normal intrauterine pregnancies sooner than with transabdominal techniques and thus to shorten the window between biochemical detection and reliable imaging within the uterus.

Published work by this author as well as others seems to indicate that with high-frequency endovaginal ultrasound probes, normal intrauterine pregnancies will be imaged when the hCG level is greater than approximately 1,025 mIU/ml (IRP). In the author's study, 235 patients (all less than or equal to 7 weeks from the last menstrual period and either requesting pregnancy testing or pregnancy termination) were scanned using a 5-MHz endovaginal probe. None of the patients had any vaginal bleeding. Serum hCG levels were obtained when no sac was seen on endovaginal scan or a sac was visualized but was less than or equal to 1.0-cm maximal sac diameter. The initial pilot study revealed that 20 patients whose maximal sac diameter was greater than 1.0 cm on endovaginal scan all had hCG levels greater than 6,000 mIU/ml (IRP).

Of these patients, 154 demonstrated intrauterine sacs greater than 1.0 cm, and this finding was confirmed at the time of termination of pregnancy. Pathologic study revealed chorionic villi in all patients.

Twenty patients had intrauterine sacs between 0.5 cm and 1.0 cm. Levels of hCG ranged from 1,025–6,074 mIU/ml (IRP) (Fig. 4–8). In 41 patients, no sac was visualized. Thirty-one of them were not pregnant (hCG level less than 5 mIU/ml) and the ten that were had hCG levels ranging from 394–5,544 mIU/ml (IRP) (Table 4–1). Note that three normal pregnancies (as diagnosed by pathologic examination at the time of termination) were coexisting with multiple myomas in two and an IUD in the third (Fig. 4–9A,B).

Endovaginal Scanning Study

- 235 patients
- all ≤ 7 weeks LMP
- no vaginal bleeding
- all requesting pregnancy testing or pregnancy termination
- serum hCG levels obtained when
  1) no sac was seen on endovaginal scan
  2) sac was visualized but was ≤ 1.0 cm on endovaginal scan

This study shows that the intact fluid of a normal sac surrounded by its echogenic rind allows for its ultrasonic recognition. This is not true in abnormal situations of pregnancy (ectopics, complete or missed abortions) or in very early normal pregnancies in uteri with heterogenous echoes (myomas, IUDs). Thus endovaginal ultrasound can be a reliable way of detecting *normal* intrauterine pregnancies in *normal* uteri when the sac size exceeds 0.4 cm maximal diameter or when the serum hCG level exceeds 1,025 mIU/ml (IRP).

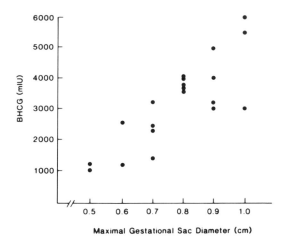

Fig. 4–8. Beta-hCG levels of 20 intrauterine pregnancies with maximal sac diameter between 0.5 cm and 1.0 cm.

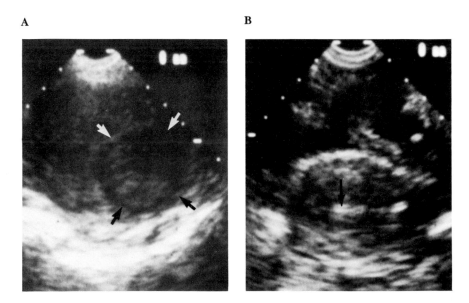

Fig. 4–9. (A) Endovaginal scan of patient with a beta-hCG level of 3,944 mIU/ml (IRP). No gestational sac was imaged. There were multiple myomas (arrows). Suction curettage revealed normal-appearing chorionic villi. **(B)** Endovaginal scan of pregnant patient with a beta-hCG level of 2,007 mIU/ml (IRP). Centrally located IUD is visualized (arrow). No gestational sac was seen. Suction curettage revealed normal-appearing placental tissue.

TABLE 4-1. Ten Patients With Biochemical Evidence of Pregnancy in Whom No Evidence on an Intrauterine Sac Was Seen With Endovaginal Ultrasound

Patient no.	hCG level at time of scan (mIU/ml)	Findings on endovaginal scan	Follow-up	Pathology report	Final diagnosis
1	1,976	No intrauterine sac	Suction D&C	Necrotic chorionic villi	Missed abortion
2	708	No sac seen	Repeat hCG = 547; suction D&C 1 week later	Necrotic chorionic villi	Missed abortion
3	3,947	No sac seen	Suction D&C	Necrotic chorionic villi	Missed abortion
4	1,972	No sac seen	Suction D&C; repeat hCG=445 and 5 mIU at 48 and 168 hours, respectively	Necrotic decidua	Complete abortion, possibly tubal
5	394	No sac seen	Repeat hCG = 19 at 1 week and 5 at 2 weeks		Complete abortion, possibly tubal
6	6,000	No IUG, extrauterine sac	Suction D&C	Decidua only; no necrosis	Laparotomy revealed left ectopic pregnancy
7	4,125	Decidual cast	Suction D&C	Decidua only; no necrosis	Laparotomy revealed right ectopic pregnancy
8	5,544	Fibroid uterus, no IUG	Suction D&C	Normal chorionic villi	Normal pregnancy, fibroid uterus
9	3,944	Fibroid uterus, no IUG	Suction D&C	Normal chorionic villi	Normal pregnancy, fibroid uterus
10	2,007	No sac seen, IUD	Suction D&C	Normal chorionic villi	Normal pregnancy, coexisting IUD

YOLK SAC

After the appearance of the gestational sac, the next structure visible sonographically is the yolk sac, which, as already mentioned, has been present since the blastocyst stage and implantation. We are first able to image it at about 3–3½ weeks postconception. It is fetal in origin and is extra-amniotic (a fact better illustrated later).

The yolk sac is a fairly constant round structure about 4 mm in diameter, with a thin but bright echogenic rim around a sonolucent center (Fig. 4–10). It will remain quite constant until about 10 weeks. As the gestational sac and embryo grow, the yolk sac may become sonographically obscured, and as the pregnancy advances it will regress to a remnant that becomes incorporated beneath the amnion. The only significance to us as sonographers or clinicians is that the yolk sac is an ultrasound landmark that

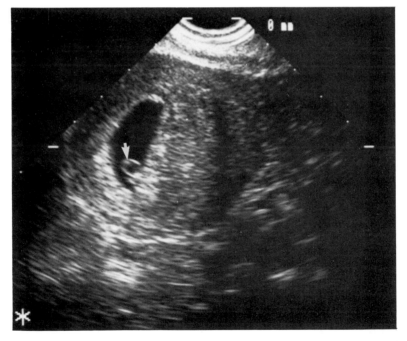

Fig. 4–10. Endovaginal scan showing yolk sac contained within an early gestational sac. Note its bright echogenic rim (arrow) around a sonolucent interior.

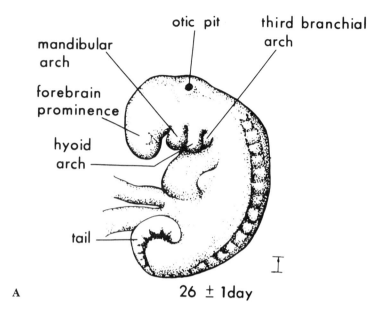

otic pit

third branchial arch

mandibular arch

forebrain prominence

hyoid arch

tail

A

26 ± 1day

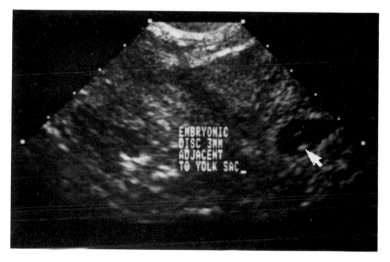

B

Fig. 4–11. (A) Drawing of embryo at approximately 26 days postconception. The entire embryonic disc measures 3 mm at this point. **(B)** Endovaginal ultrasound at the same stage as the drawing in **A**. Note 3-mm embryonic disc (arrow) as bright echogenic structure adjacent to yolk sac. Fetal cardiac activity can be demonstrated at this point with m-mode capability. (Drawing reproduced with permission from Keith L. Moore, *The Developing Human,* 4th ed. Philadelphia, W.B. Saunders Co., 1988.)

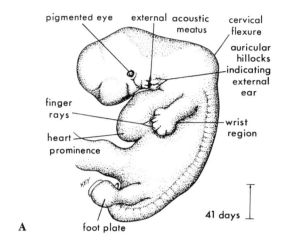

A

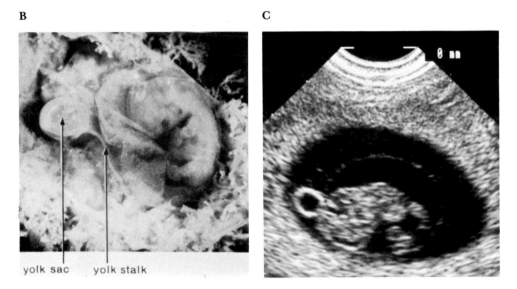

B   C

yolk sac   yolk stalk

Fig. 4-12. (A) Drawing of fetus at 8 weeks LMP. **(B)** Photograph of an embryo at the same stage as the drawing in A. Note the relationship of the yolk sac and yolk stalk outside the amniotic cavity containing the embryo. **(C)** Endovaginal ultrasound at the same time period as **A** and **B.** The embryo is just beginning to unfold. It is contained within the amnion, which has not yet fused with chorion. Yolk sac is seen to be extra-amniotic. (**A** and **B** reproduced with permission from Keith L. Moore, *The Developing Human*, 4th ed. Philadelphia, W.B. Saunders Co., 1988.)

precedes our ability to see the embryo by about one-half to one week. A normal image is reassuring. Some pathologic significance has been attached to a yolk sac that appears enlarged, malformed, or "free-floating."

EMBRYONIC POLE

The first evidence of embryonic development definitively separate from the yolk sac was previously referred to as a "fetal pole," which we prefer to label an "embryonic pole." As previously mentioned, it is usually seen 3–7 days after visualization of the yolk sac and appears as a small echogenic focus. Virtually as early as one sees an embryonic pole, one will be able to demonstrate cardiac activity. This is not surprising, since embryologically we know that before the end of the third week postconception the paired endocardial heart tubes have fused and that by the 21st day this primitive heart has lined up with blood vessels in the embryo, the connecting stalk, the chorion, and the yolk sac to form a primitive cardiovascular system. Thus the cardiovascular system is the first organ system to reach a functional state. Some endovaginal probes with m-mode capability can definitively document cardiac activity. However, the ability to "eyeball" cardiac activity will depend on the resolution of the equipment and the visual acuity of the examiner (see further discussion in the section on missed abortion in Chapter 5).

Although embryologically there is a great deal of differentiation in the 2–5-mm embryo, we are not able to appreciate fine detail at this stage with current equipment (Fig. 4–11A,B). At this point the embryo grows about 1 mm per day. By the time the crown rump length is 1.4 cm (about 41 days postconception), we can clearly see the embryo beginning to unfold. The head accounts for about one-half its size (Fig. 4–12A–C).

We must comment here on conceptual age versus menstrual age. Clinically we are all too familar with the uncertainty of menstrual data. Even in patients with reliable menstrual data, there will be up to several days variation in when ovulation occurs. Thus, we should avoid being dogmatic about when which anatomic landmarks appear; there must be leeway of at least one-half a week. As in vitro fertilization becomes common and more data are generated from cases in which exact time of conception is known, then perhaps dating of landmarks will become more precise. Of course, we do not know if the in vitro process might not slightly alter the embryologic time course. Furthermore, no one knows absolutely how much variation on the "average" there may be for the embryogenesis process in general.

The transition from embryo to fetus is not abrupt. The word *fetus* (from the Latin for "offspring") is used when development has progressed far enough to give the appearance of a human being. *Embryo* is from the Greek and defines an organism in the early stages of development, for example, before metamorphosis. Thus by the end of the seventh conceptual week, as we shall see in Chapter 6, we have certainly entered the fetal period.

SUGGESTED READINGS

Goldstein SR. Early pregnancy ultrasound: A new look with the endovaginal probe. Contemp Ob Gyn 31:54, 1988.

Goldstein SR, et al. Very early pregnancy detection with endovaginal ultrasound. Obstet Gynecol 72:200–204, 1988.

Jeanty P, Romero R. Obstetrical Ultrasound. New York: McGraw Hill, 1984.

Kadar N, Caldwell BV, Romero R. A method of screening for ectopic pregnancy and its indications. Obstet Gynecol 58:156–161, 1981.

Kadar N, DeVore G, Romero R. Discriminatory hCG zone: Its use in the sonographic evaluation for ectopic pregnancy. Obstet Gynecol 58:156–161, 1981.

Moore KL. The Developing Human, Ed 4. Philadelphia: WB Saunders and Company, 1988.

Nyberg DA, Laing FC, Filly RA, et al. Ultrasound differentiation of the gestational sac of early pregnancy from the psuedo-gestational sac of ectopic pregnancy. Radiology 146:755–759, 1983.

Shenker L, Astle C, Reed K, et al. Embryonic heart rates before the seventh week of pregnancy. J Reprod Med 31:333, 1986.

Timor-Tritsch IE, et al. Review of transvaginal ultrasonography. Ultrasound 6:1, 1988.

Chapter 5

Pregnancy II:
Something Is Wrong

In 1985 the National Institutes of Health (NIH) held a consensus panel to look into questions of safety with respect to ultrasonography in pregnancy. Although the panel found no evidence of any harmful effects of diagnostic ultrasound in pregnancy, it could not *prove* that ultrasound was indeed safe. Thus the panel concluded there should be some clinical indication for an obstetrical ultrasound exam and provided more than two dozen valid indications.

Early pregnancy endovaginal ultrasound employs higher frequencies in closer proximity to structures being studied. This is done at a time of ongoing organogenesis. Therefore any theoretical concerns about bioeffects will be at least as pertinent if not more so in endovaginal first-trimester scanning. Thus the purpose of this chapter is to reiterate the clinical situations that are appropriate indications for first-trimester endovaginal ultrasound scanning and to present the expected ultrasound findings.

THREATENED ABORTION

Threatened abortion is a clinical term. It is defined as a pregnancy of less than 20 weeks with vaginal bleeding and a closed cervical os. It is undoubtedly the most common indication for first-trimester ultrasound request.

Perhaps as many as one-half of such patients will show a normal-appearing intrauterine gestation (findings dependent on the age of gestation), with no obvious reason for or source of the clinically apparent vaginal bleeding. In such cases ultrasound may not provide the clinician with a cause for the vaginal bleeding, but the finding of a normal gestation may be extremely reassuring. A positive fetal heart after 8 weeks last menstrual period (LMP) is associated with a continuation rate as high as 95% for that pregnancy.

Subchorionic Hemorrhage

Researchers have long attempted to find parameters both ultrasonagraphically and biochemically to enhance our prognostic predictability in cases of threatened abortion. Investigators have looked at various biochemical markers, including hCG, serum progesterone, and even serum human placental lactogen (HPL) levels. Previously, the presence of fetal heart was found to be associated with approximately 85–90% continuation rate. This ultrasound finding seemed to be a better prognosticator than any of the biochemical markers mentioned above.

More recently the finding of subchorionic bleeding has enhanced our prognosticating ability in cases of threatened abortion. Subchorionic hemorrhage is identified as a crescent-shaped sonolucent collection outside of the gestational sac (Fig. 5–1). In the original description of the condition, patients with positive fetal heart activity and no evidence of any subchorionic bleeding had a pregnancy continuation rate that approached 100%. In those patients with a positive fetal heart along with evidence of subchorionic bleeding, the continuation rate seemed to be in the range of 70%. There appeared to be no good correlation between the size and amount of subchorionic blood and the eventual outcome. Subchorionic bleeding will manifest in approximately 20% of cases of threatened abortion with demonstrated fetal viability. Endovaginal ultrasound is a quick and convenient way to examine patients who have bleeding in the first trimester of pregnancy.

Embryonic Resorption

Previously, blighted ovum and missed abortion were considered separate clinical and ultrasonagraphic entities. Actually, in some cases they may represent the same process, occurring at different

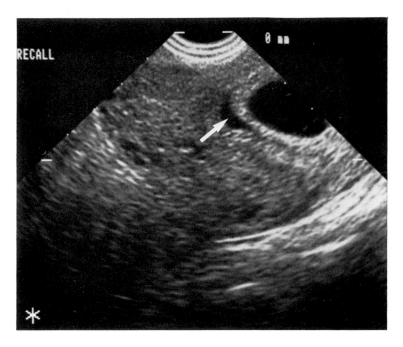

Fig. 5-1. Endovaginal scan of patient at 7 weeks last menstrual period (LMP) who presented clinically with vaginal bleeding (i.e., threatened abortion). Scan revealed a normal gestational sac with embryo and cardiac activity (not seen in this scanning plane). Note subchorionic hemorrhage (arrow) represented by crescent-shaped sonolucency outside the gestational sac.

times in the first trimester. Indeed there may be embryonic development to some point followed by resorption of the embryo. This is probably the mechanism involved in the so-called "vanishing twin" (see below).

Blighted Ovum

Previously thought of as an anembryonic pregnancy, this condition may actually represent very early embryonic resorption such that no identifiable embryo is seen within the gestational sac. The previous ultrasound definition (Fig. 5-2) was primarily a large sac (>25 mm mean sac diameter) without evidence of an embryo and a sac with markedly distorted shape. Endovaginal ultrasound will undoubtedly change this definition. It remains to

---

Defining Blighted Ovum

Anembryonic pregnancy vs embryonic resorption

Previous ultrasound definition

      Large sac (>25 mm mean sac diameter) without embryo

      Distorted shape

Endovaginal ultrasound definition

      Sac (? size) without yolk sac/embryo

---

be seen, however, at what size gestational sac the lack of a visible yolk sac/embryo will be pathognomonic of pregnancy failure. The real question is not how early one can see a yolk sac or embryo within the gestational sac but rather how late in the pregnancy or at what size can the sac grow without obvious yolk sac or embryo formation before one can be definite about the nonviability of that pregnancy.

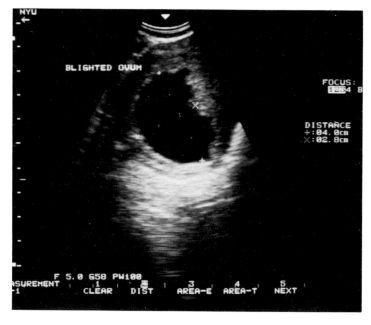

Fig. 5-2. Endovaginal scan revealing large irregularly shaped gestational sac. Patient had clinical history of spotting. No recognizable embryonic structure was seen. Such a "blighted ovum," previously thought to be an anembryonic pregnancy, may actually represent varying degrees of embryonic resorption. The sac, marked by calipers, measures 4.0×2.8 cm.

As more studies appear in the literature concerning the sac size at which lack of embryonic development represents nonviable pregnancy, the beginner in endovaginal ultrasound should exercise extreme caution. Remember, these are very early pregnancies. Spontaneous abortion from such pregnancies is rarely associated with extraordinary blood loss and/or infection. If any doubt exists, serial ultrasound scan is an appropriate clinical course to follow. It is our experience that very early gestational sacs, when normal, are fairly round and consistent in shape. We take a maximal sac diameter measurement. Some investigators who report their work in "mean sac diameters" are taking three measurements from two pictures at perfect right angles to each other. Such views may not always be available to the endovaginal sonographer. In a desired pregnancy that may be borderline in appearance, always give the pregnancy the benefit of the doubt and suggest repeat ultrasound examination in ½–1 week.

Missed Abortion

Missed abortion is defined as a nonviable pregnancy that has not yet been passed. Previously it was felt that a gestation may lose viability from 1–4 weeks prior to spontaneous passage. Virtually 95% of all pregnancies will pass spontaneously within 4 weeks of loss of viability.

The previous ultrasound definition of a missed abortion (Fig. 5–3) was a crown rump length (CRL) of >15 mm with no discernible fetal heart motion. Once again, endovaginal ultrasound will markedly modify this definition. As discussed in the previous chapter, as soon as one can see a recognizable embryonic

---

Defining Missed Abortion

  Nonviable pregnancy not yet passed
  Previous ultrasound definition
      CRL >15 mm with no fetal heart motion
  Endovaginal ultrasound definition
      Recognizable embryonic pole without cardiac activity???

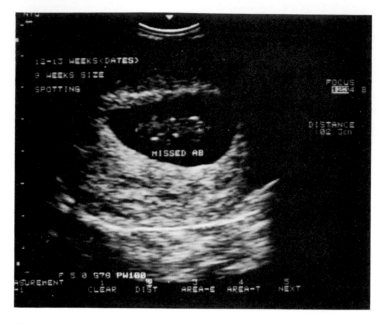

Fig. 5–3. Scan revealing embryo with crown rump length of 2.2 cm without any fetal cardiac activity. Patient was 13 weeks LMP. Clinical history consisted of vaginal spotting and pelvic exam revealing uterine size small for dates.

pole, fetal cardiac activity can be expected. However, without m-mode capability, the definitive diagnosis of cardiac activity in very small embryonic structures will depend on the resolution of the equipment and the visual acuity of the examiner. Once again caution must be emphasized. If a small embryonic structure separate from the yolk sac is visualized but no definitive cardiac activity is recognized, it is suggested that the patient be rescanned in ½–1 week.

Vanishing Twin

There is a generally accepted twinning rate of approximately 1 in 80 liveborn pregnancies. It has been reported that approximately 70% of twin gestations diagnosed at 10 weeks will be singletons at term. This is the basis for the so-called vanishing twin (Fig. 5–4). The mechanism for this embryological/fetal resorption in which twins may become a singleton may indeed be

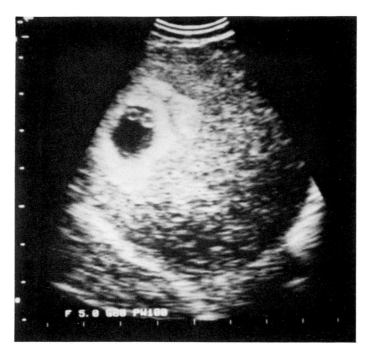

Fig. 5-4. Endovaginal scan at 5.5 weeks LMP. Two distinct yolk sacs are seen within a single gestational sac. One small embryonic pole with cardiac activity was noted. Follow-up scan in 2 weeks revealed a single gestational sac with a single viable embryo whose CRL measured 1.3 cm. This case of embryonic resorption is an example of the "vanishing twin."

the same as that for the singleton that becomes a "blighted ovum."

Sonographically, the vanishing twin must be distinguished from subchorionic hemorrhage, which may be a difficult task. The true vanishing twin may still exhibit some of the trophoblastic decidual reaction that can help to distinguish it from cases of subchorionic bleeding (Fig. 5-5A,B).

Ectopic Pregnancy

Many cases of threatened abortion will include as part of their differential diagnosis "r/o ectopic pregnancy." This is such an important topic that it will be considered in its own chapter (see Chapter 8). Here it will suffice to say that endovaginal ultrasound

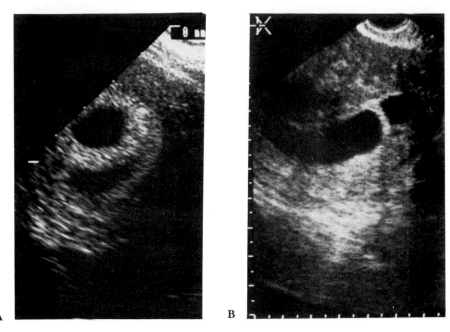

A   B

Fig. 5-5. (**A**) Patient at 6 weeks LMP with vaginal spotting. Superiorly one notes a normal-appearing gestational sac that is very round, with well-developed trophoblastic decidual reaction. Beneath it there is a slightly compressed chorionic cavity whose trophoblastic decidual reaction is less prominent. This second gestational sac, which is in the process of "vanishing," could not be imaged at follow-up scan 2 weeks later. The normal gestational sac showed appropriate interval growth during that time. (**B**) A 7.5-week LMP normal gestational sac that had a viable embryo within. Adjacent sonolucent area in this patient with clinical history of spotting represents subchorionic hemorrhage. This should not be mistaken for a "vanishing twin."

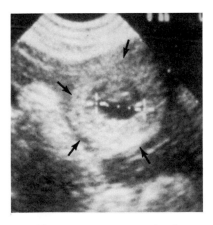

Fig. 5-6. The more normal in appearance a gestation is regardless of its location, the more likely it will be imaged with ultrasound techniques. This is an obvious (arrows) extrauterine gestational sac that contains an embryonic pole with fetal cardiac activity within it. Definitive diagnosis here makes diagnostic laparoscopy unnecessary.

scanning will allow us to diagnose ectopic pregnancy earlier and more reliably, in the following ways:

1. A higher percentage of ectopics will be definitively identified with endovaginal scanning techniques (Fig. 5–6).
2. Earlier and more reliable recognition of intrauterine pregnancy will "rule out" ectopic. This will occur more reliably and earlier in gestation, thus decreasing unnecessary surgical procedures and providing reassurance in high-risk cases.
3. Pretermination screening with ultrasound can identify unsuspected ectopic pregnancies at the time of elective terminations (see Chapter 9).

SIZE-DATES DISCREPANCY

Pregnancy Dating

Sonographically, the CRL has been the most accurate method of dating a pregnancy in the first trimester. Tables relating crown rump length and gestational age are readily available and are programmed into the software of much of the ultrasound equipment currently being utilized. A quick rule of thumb is to add 6.5 to the crown rump length in cm to obtain the number of menstrual weeks. Previously common errors in measuring the CRL were: 1) failure to identify the longest fetal diameter; 2) including lower limbs; 3) including yolk sac; and 4) including a portion of uterine wall. The kind of resolution that previous ultrasound scanners afforded resulted in the compilation of the above-mentioned list. With endovaginal scanning techniques, there is very little uncertainty as to the precise measurement of the crown rump length for dating (Fig. 5–7A,B).

It should be kept in mind, however, that pregnancy dating is not a significant problem in patients who present early in the first trimester. Even with old traditional transabdominal techniques, the crown rump length was accurate to within approximately ½ week. Although endovaginal ultrasound will result in less error in measuring crown rump length, the actual change in pregnancy dating can be expected to be small and is not likely to have the tremendous clinical significance that ultrasonographically derived pregnancy dating can provide in those obstetrical patients who are late registrants and who have uncertain menstrual histories.

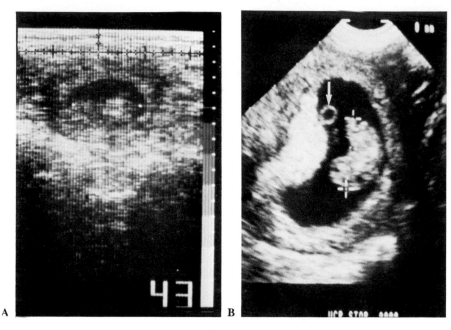

Fig. 5-7. (**A**) Old linear array real-time scan depicting crown rump length at 11 weeks. Note lack of clarity of anatomical landmarks for positioning of electronic calipers to measure CRL (43 mm). (**B**) Endovaginal scan at 9 weeks LMP. Calipers depict crown rump length as 23 mm. Note yolk sac (arrow) adjacent to fetus. Note the increased precision for measuring CRL that endovaginal scanning provides.

Inaccurate Dates

Accurate pregnancy dating even in the first trimester is especially important for patients anticipating prenatal genetic diagnosis (amniocentesis, chorion villous sampling, or maternal serum alpha-fetoprotein [AFP] testing). It will be equally important when cervical circlage is anticipated, if elective repeat cesarean section is planned, or if the pregnancy is to be voluntarily terminated (see Chapter 9).

Coexisting Myomas

Myomas of the uterus coexisting with a first-trimester gestation are another common cause for a size-dates discrepancy. Endovaginal ultrasound allows a quick and efficient way of accurately dating such pregnancies, the importance of which has been previously discussed. In addition, in those patients electing voluntary termination, the location of fibroid changes relative to the location of the gestational sac and the endocervical canal will be extremely important in enhancing the safety of the suction curettage procedure.

Coexisting myomas must be distinguished from focal myometrial contractions, which may appear fibroid-like sonographically. They tend to be highly symmetrical and to indent the gestational sac (Fig. 5–8A,B). They are of clinical significance in patients about to undergo a chorion villous sampling procedure. When present, the patient may get off the table and ambulate for approximately 15 minutes, and most often such focal myometrial contractions will dissipate.

A   B

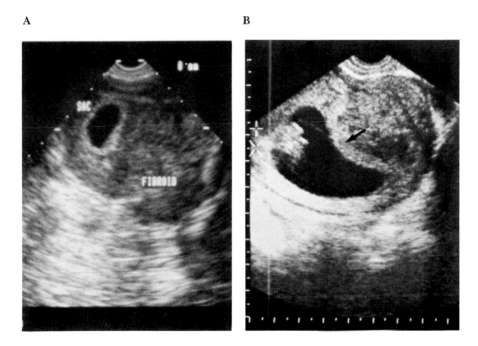

Fig. 5–8. (A) Patient at 6.5 weeks LMP whose uterus on clinical exam was 13–14 weeks size. Endovaginal scan clearly shows gestational sac, corroborating menstrual data with presence of coexisting fibroid. (B) Endosonographic appearance of a focal myometrial contraction in a pregnancy of 9 weeks LMP. The focal contraction causes an indentation of the gestational sac (arrow). These are quite common and short-lived. If present prior to chorion villous sampling, one should allow the patient to get off the examining table to ambulate for 15–20 minutes. The scan is then repeated.

Multiple Gestation

Multiple gestations are another source of size-dates discrepancy in the first trimester (Fig. 5–9). It is important that the sonographer carefully view the entire uterus to accurately assess the number of gestations present. Occasionally, uterine malformation such as a septated uterus can, in certain scanning planes, appear as a multiple gestation (Fig. 5–10A,B). Once again the examiner must carefully assess the entire uterine contents in multiple planes.

Hydatidiform Mole

Hydatidiform mole will result in a classic ultrasound appearance of multiple small sonolucent areas corresponding to the

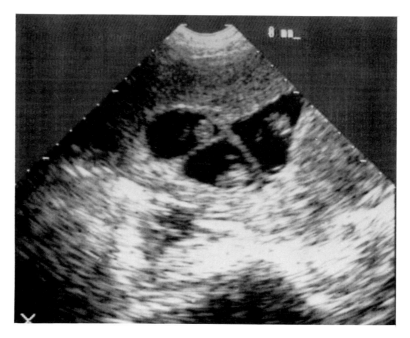

Fig. 5–9. Endovaginal scan revealing triplets at 8 weeks LMP. With increasing ovulation induction and in vitro fertilization, the incidence of multiple gestations is increasing. As the number of gestational sacs increases, it becomes more difficult to definitively count the number present. It may take considerable skill and time when more than four sacs are present.

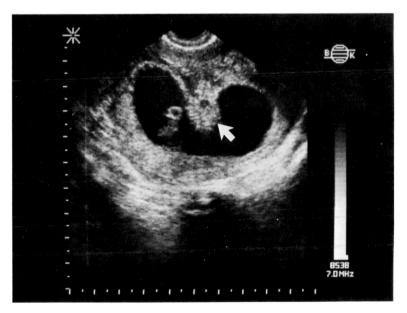

Fig. 5-10. (**A**) Patient at 9.5 weeks LMP. In this scanning plane there appear to be twin gestational sacs (arrows). (**B**) On more careful scanning of the patient in **A**, it became obvious that this was a single gestation wrapped around a uterine septum (arrow). The operator must carefully scan the entire uterus in cases of suspected multiple gestation in order to exclude the artifacts that uterine anomalies can cause.

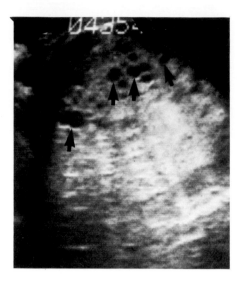

Fig. 5–11. Endovaginal scan showing classic appearance of hydatidiform mole. Note the multiple sonolucent areas (arrows) corresponding to the hydropic grape-like structures that one typically sees on gross examination of pathologic tissue.

"grape-like" vesicles that one sees on gross pathologic examination (Fig. 5–11). Rarely are such changes sonographically apparent prior to 10 weeks menstrual age. This is because the trophoblastic proliferation and hydropic changes seen grossly with hydatidiform mole are not manifest prior to this time.

Pregnancy Failure

As previously mentioned, cases of pregnancy failure (embryonic resorption) can be a major cause of the "small-for-dates" uterus.

In some of the examples given in this chapter, the tremendous advantage of endovaginal ultrasound stems from the higher resolution (even with magnification) that results from the probes being of higher frequency and in closer proximity to the structures being imaged. In other examples, the main advantage is in the immense saving of time, either because the clinician can perform the sonography at the time of pelvic examination or because the exam can be done with an empty bladder, even in the radiologic suite.

SUGGESTED READINGS

Bernard KG, Cooperberg PL. Sonographic differentiation between blighted ovum and early viable pregnancy. Am J Roentgenol 144:597–601, 1985.

Callen PW. Ultrasonography in Obstetrics and Gynecology. Philadelphia: WB Saunders and Company, 1983.

Finberg HJ, Birnholz JC. Ultrasound observation in multiple gestation with first trimester bleeding: The blighted twin. Radiology 132:137–142, 1979.

Goldstein SR, et al. Subchorionic bleeding in threatened abortion: Sonographic findings and significance. Am J Roentgenol 141:975–978, 1983.

Goldstein SR. Early pregnancy ultrasound: A new look with the endovaginal probe. Contemp Ob Gyn 31:54, 1988.

Jeanty P, Romero R. Obstetrical Ultrasound. New York: McGraw Hill, 1984.

Kadar N, Caldwell BV, Romero R. A method of screening for ectopic pregnancy and its indications. Obstet Gynecol 58:162–166, 1981.

Kadar N, DeVore G, Romero R. Discriminatory hCG zone: Its use in the sonographic evaluation for ectopic pregnancy. Obstet Gynecol 58:156–161, 1981.

Mendelson EB, Bohm-Velez N. Transvaginal sonography assesses early pregnancy. Diagn Imaging 9:243–248, 1987.

Nyberg D, Filly R, Filho D, et al. Abnormal pregacy: Early diagnosis by ultrasound and serum chorionic gonadotropin levels. Radiology 158:393–396, 1986.

Nyberg DA, Laing FC, Filly RA, et al. Ultrasound differentiation of the gestational sac of early pregnancy from the psuedo-gestational sac of ectopic pregnancy. Radiology 146:755–759, 1983.

Romero R, Kadar N, Jeanty P, et al. Diagnosis of ectopic pregnancy: Value of the discriminatory human chorionic gonadotropin zone. Obstet Gynecol 66:357–360, 1985.

Chapter 6

Pregnancy III:
Fetus, First Trimester

As a result of the higher frequency of endovaginal probes and the increased resolution that results, even with magnification, fetal anatomical structures are imaged at gestational ages never before possible. From 10–14 weeks LMP, endovaginal images are of high quality and may indeed surpass even the finest currently available traditional abdominal scanners. However, by this time the portion of the fetus at interest can often be out of the effective focal range of the endovaginal probe. If the fetal part of interest is close to the lower uterine segment it may well be imaged, but unfortunately this will not always be the case.

The most exciting fetal time frame for endovaginal ultrasound is in the 8–10-week LMP range. This is when endovaginal ultrasound will prove its superior usefulness through its consistent ability to image structures previously unnoticed with the traditional transabdominal technique.

FETAL ANATOMY

Since the very beginnings of obstetrical ultrasound, the "midline echo" has been the most important intracranial structure. It appears as a bright, linear echogenic structure in the midportion of the head. It serves as one of the principle landmarks for measuring the biparietal diameter (BPD), which was the first fetal measurement to be related to gestational age. The BPD is not traditionally employed until it reaches approximately 2.0 cm at 12 weeks LMP. Using endovaginal techniques, the midline echo (and thus a BPD measurement) can often be obtained in the range of 9–10 weeks LMP (Fig. 6–1).

There are other intracranial landmarks more recently described than the BPD that can also be imaged by the tenth week LMP. They include the orbits (Figs. 6–2, 6–3), the choroid plexus (which appears on both sides of the midline as a half-heart-shaped echogenic structure [Fig. 6–4]), and the recently described rhombencephalon, which appears as a sonolucent structure in the posterior aspect of the fetal cranium at about 8–10 weeks LMP. After the 11th menstrual week, this structure will evolve into the normal fourth ventricle (Fig. 6–5).

Skeletal Findings

Facial bones, including maxillary sinuses, maxilla, and mandible, can be imaged. Limb girdles, including the shoulder and

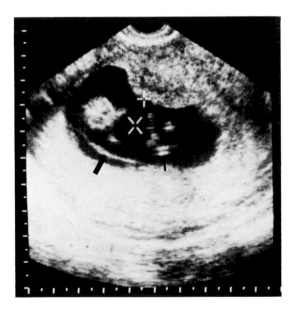

Fig. 6–1. The echogenicity of the midline echo is clearly seen in the head of this fetus at 10 weeks LMP. The biparietal diameter as measured by the calipers (which were then moved so as not to obscure the landmarks involved) is 11 mm. In this scanning plane we also see a portion of fetal femur (small arrow). In addition, chorion and amnion have not yet fused (large arrow).

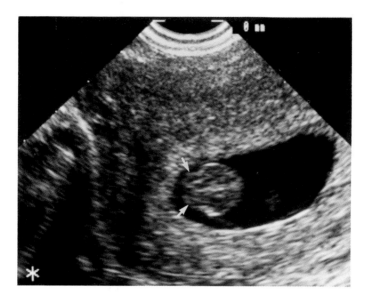

Fig. 6-2. The binocular distance is easily seen here in the anterior portion (arrows) of this transverse section of fetal head at 10 weeks LMP.

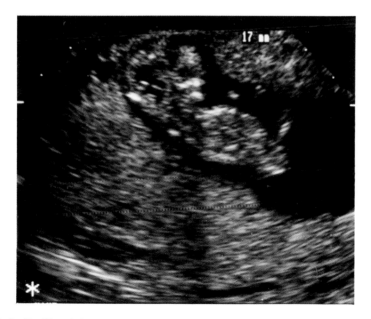

Fig. 6-3. Profile of the same fetus clearly showing the eye in long axis. In addition, the well-demarcated maxilla and mandible are seen.

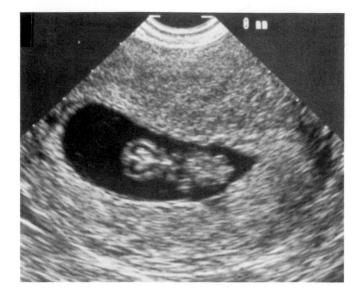

Fig. 6-4. Endovaginal scan at 9.5 weeks LMP clearly showing echogenic choroid plexus within the fetal head.

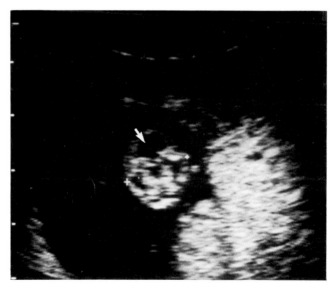

Fig. 6-5. Endovaginal scan at 10 weeks LMP (BPD = 1.2) clearly showing large sonolucent structure in the posterior aspect of the fetal cranium (arrow), which is the rhombencephalon. This will evolve into the fourth ventricle.

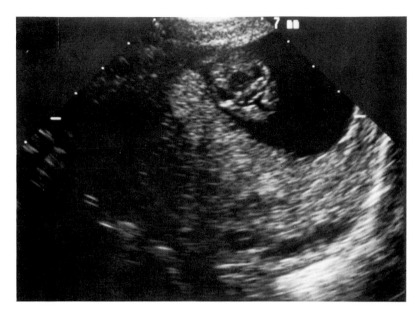

Fig. 6-6. Coronal cut of the fetal head at 9.5 weeks showing maxillary sinuses as well as small portion of fetal maxilla.

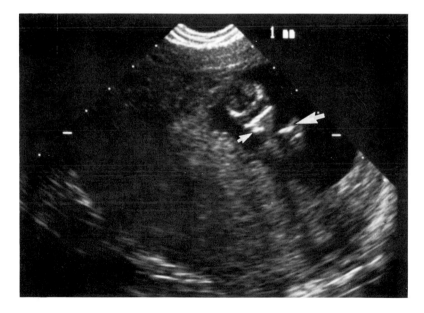

Fig. 6-7. Same fetus as in Figure 6-6. Maxilla, portion of mandible (small arrow), and left shoulder girdle (large arrow) are noted.

pelvic regions, are easily identified (Figs. 6–6, 6–7, 6–8), and limb buds and developing extremities are visualized with excellent precision (Figs. 6–9, 6–10, 6–11). The spine at 9–10 weeks LMP does not cause acoustic shadowing. This is probably a result of insufficient calcification and ossification at this early stage of development (Fig. 6–12).

Fetal Abdomen

Fetal stomach is easily recognized by its sonolucent appearance when full (Fig. 6–13). Normal fetal kidneys are echogenic and can be more difficult to image at this early stage of gestation. There is a physiological herniation of gut that occurs between 7 and 9 weeks LMP. The midgut herniates through the yolk stalk, undergoes a 270° rotation, and re-enters the abdominal cavity (Fig. 6–14). By 10 weeks, however, normal insertion of the umbilical cord into the abdomen can be imaged (Fig. 6–15).

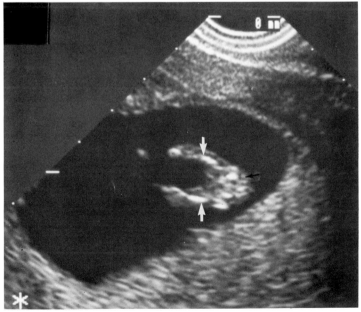

Fig. 6–8. Fetal ilium and ischium (small arrow) leading into fetal femurs (large arrows) seen here at 10 weeks LMP.

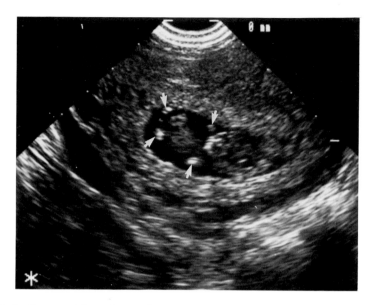

Fig. 6–9. Fetus at 9.5 weeks LMP clearly showing the development of all four limb buds (arrows). Echogenicity is portion of fetal mandible.

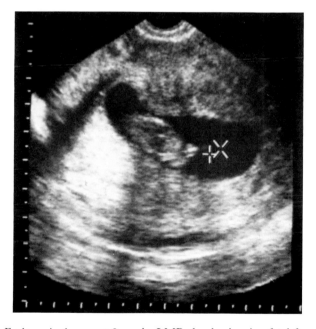

Fig. 6–10. Endovaginal scan at 9 weeks LMP clearly showing fetal femur as well as fetal tibia. Femur length here measures 4 mm, and calipers have been displaced appropriately so as not to obscure the landmarks they are measuring.

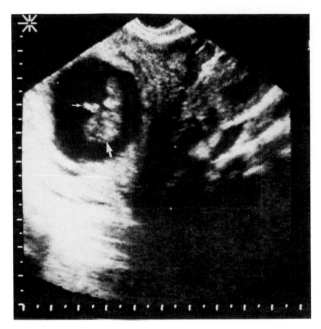

Fig. 6–11. Fetus at 9 weeks showing fetal arms (small arrow). Note portion of fetal trunk distally (large arrow).

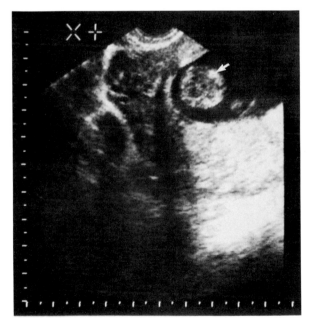

Fig. 6–12. Endovaginal scan depicting cross section of fetal abdomen at 9 weeks LMP. Abdominal diameter here is 8 mm. The echogenic fetal spine is identified (arrow). There is no acoustic shadowing, probably from insufficient calcification this early in pregnancy.

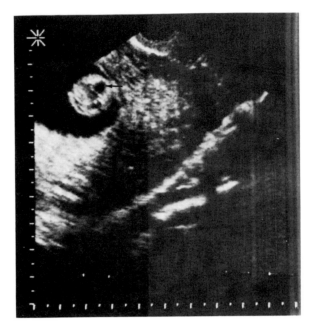

Fig. 6-13. Fetal abdomen in cross section at 9 weeks LMP. Round sonolucent structure seen here (arrow) is filled fetal stomach. Fetal bladder is not readily discernible at this early stage of pregnancy.

Certainly, endovaginal ultrasound offers enhanced ability to image fetal anatomy in the late first trimester, but as we have already mentioned, there are certain limitations to the technique. First, according to fetal lie, not all structures will be able to be imaged, depending on the scanning planes that one can obtain as well as on the amount of time spent. Furthermore, the amount of time spent should reflect the indication for the scan and the "index of suspicion." Remember that transducer mobility is somewhat limited by the confines of the vagina and also by the design of the transducer being employed. In addition, with the very high-frequency endovaginal probes the effective focal range may be no more than 6 cm from the transducer. Thus by the late first trimester many of the desired anatomical structures may be out of the field of vision of the examiner.

It remains to be seen at what gestational age various fetal anomalies will be diagnosable with absolute reliability by endovaginal ultrasound. Certainly, however, there is great promise for

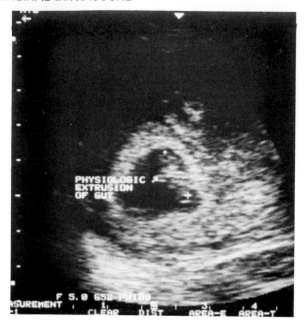

Fig. 6–14. Fetus at 8 weeks LMP demonstrating physiological herniation of gut (arrow), which will undergo a 270° rotation before re-entering the abdominal cavity.

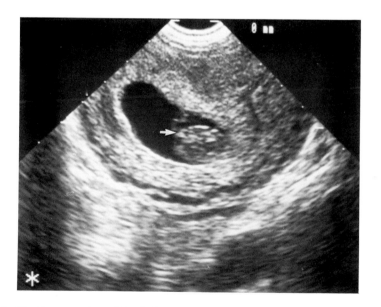

Fig. 6–15. Cross section of fetal abdomen at 10 weeks LMP. Note normal insertion of umbilical cord (arrow). All of the herniated midgut has re-entered the peritoneal cavity by this time.

earlier diagnosis of fetal anomalies previously not appreciated until well into the second trimester.

SUGGESTED READINGS

Callen PW. Ultrasonography in Obstetrics and Gynecology. Philadelphia: WB Saunders and Company, 1983.

Goldstein SR. Early pregnancy ultrasound: A new look with the endovaginal probe. Contemp Ob Gyn 31:54, 1988.

Jeanty P, Romero R. Obstetrical Ultrasound. New York: McGraw Hill, 1984.

Mendelson EB, Bohm-Velez M. Diagn Imaging November, 1987, p 244.

Moore KL. The Developing Human, Ed 4. Philadelphia: WB Saunders and Company, 1988.

Timor-Tritsch IE, et al. Review of transvaginal ultrasound. Ultrasound 6:1, 1988.

Chapter 7

Pregnancy IV:
After the First Trimester

Let us begin this chapter by reiterating some basic principles for understanding the kinds of clinical situations in which endovaginal ultrasound can be extremely helpful, and the kinds in which its value is limited. Remember that higher frequency transducers and closer proximity to the structures studied allow greater resolution, even at high magnification. However, this results in a shorter depth of the field of vision.

In addition, the fact that the endovaginal scan is done with an empty urinary bladder will save time, will lead to better acceptance by patients, and, most important, will allow the exam to be performed by the clinician in his/her office at the time of pelvic examination. However, when the urinary bladder is empty there is no acoustic window to enhance the transmission of sound. Also, loops of bowel and bizarre echoes that solid and liquid fecal matter produce will not be pushed cephalad. This means the clinician needs to reorient his sonographic "eye" for the type and format of images produced by endovaginal techniques.

For these reasons, after we leave the first trimester of pregnancy, the endovaginal technique is mainly limited to clinical situations calling for imaging of the cervix and the region near and around the cervix and lower uterine segment.

ENDOCERVICAL CANAL

The normal length of the endocervical canal will have considerable variation. This may be accounted for by individual biologic variation, parity, previous surgery, etc. The canal is sonolucent (Fig. 7–1), presumably from endocervical mucus. In the nonpregnant state as well as in the normal pregnant state, the canal is quite thin (Figs. 7–2, 7–3).

HABITUAL ABORTER (SECOND TRIMESTER)

Although first-trimester habitual abortion may have a myriad of causes, the etiological factors in the second trimester are more limited. The best known and most likely cause of midtrimester pregnancy loss is the incompetent cervical os. This is probably associated with cervical trauma, for example from previous D&C, cervical conization, laser vaporization, etc. Midtrimester pregnancy loss in the nulligravid patient, however, strongly suggests that in some patients it may represent some abnormal congenital uterine development. Furthermore, maternal ingestion of substances like diethylstilbestrol (DES) has also been implicated.

Classically, the picture is one compatible with painless cervical dilatation, premature rupture of the membranes (presumably sec-

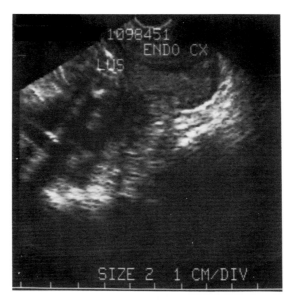

Fig. 7–1. Scan depicts normal cervix of a nonpregnant patient. The endocervical canal is seen to be thin and sonolucent (presumably from endocervical mucus). It can be traced to where it joins the lower uterine segment (LUS).

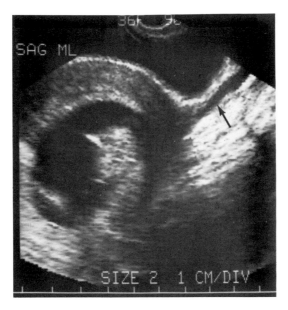

Fig. 7–2. Normal pregnancy at 10 weeks. The sonolucent endocervical canal (arrow) here is approximately 4 cm in length. A small amount of urine is seen in the bladder anteriorly.

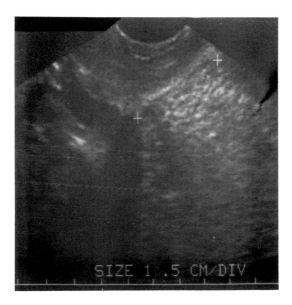

Fig. 7–3. Endocervical canal in a normal pregnancy near term. The cursors (+) show the full extent of the endocervix. It measures 1.9 cm. The sonolucent area adjacent to it is amniotic fluid surrounding a fetal part.

ondary to a low-level ascending amnionitis), and subsequent fetal loss. Frequent physical examination in patients with an index of suspicion may reveal softening and effacement of the cervix. Therapy then consists of surgical placement of a nonabsorbable suture to keep the cervix from further dilatation. The most common techniques for such a circlage procedure are the Shirodkhar or McDonald operations.

Endovaginal ultrasound can often play a useful role in the proper diagnosis of these patients. Certainly the most important aspect of diagnosis is a clinical index of suspicion, based on history. Once the index of suspicion is established, however, physical examination and endovaginal ultrasound play an important role. Endovaginal ultrasound may actually image the early signs of a loss of integrity of the internal cervical os (Fig. 7–4), and, equally as important, it may prevent a misdiagnosis.

If a diagnosis of incompetent cervical os is made and a circlage procedure is carried out, endovaginal ultrasound can be utilized to monitor the integrity of the cervix and look for any further dilatation (Figs. 7–5, 7–6).

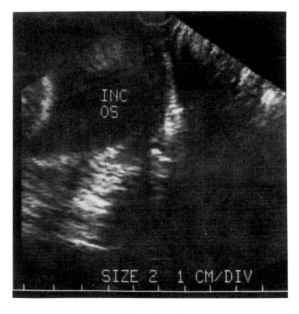

Fig. 7–4. Incompetent cervical os (INC OS). The normal configuration of the cervix and endocervical canal is absent. The amnion can be seen here ballooning in the direction of the vagina in this pregnancy at 17 weeks.

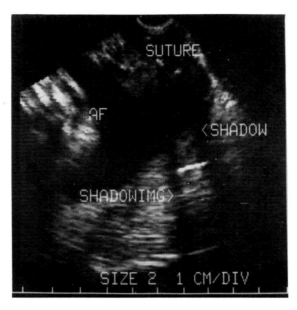

Fig. 7-5. Endovaginal scan of the patient in Figure 7-4 following a McDonald circlage procedure. Note the echogenic pieces of suture material anteriorly. The acoustic shadowing produced by this nonbiologic substance is labeled. Amniotic fluid (AF) as well as fetal parts are seen cephalad to this region.

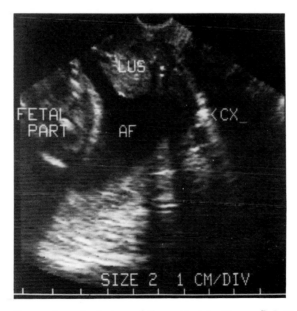

Fig. 7-6. Another endovaginal view of the patient in Figure 7-5. Note the suture material anteriorly and the acoustic shadowing that it causes. The region of the cervix is labeled (CX). Note how shortened the cervix and endocervical canal are. Once again amniotic fluid (AF) as well as fetal parts are seen on the lower uterine segment (LUS).

Another important but less common cause of habitual mid-trimester loss may be anatomical uterine defects, sometimes congenital, as in complete or partial duplication or septation of the uterus. Hysterogram in the nonpregnant state is the best diagnostic tool in such cases.

Uterine myomas can be a cause of repeated midtrimester loss. The clinical picture of such patients mimics cases of possible incompetent cervical os. Myomas may not be readily appreciated on routine pelvic examination. Endovaginal ultrasound prior to any contemplated circlage can help rule out myomas and prevent an incorrect surgical procedure (Figs. 7-7, 7-8).

PREMATURE LABOR

Premature labor remains a major source of perinatal morbidity and mortality. Earlier diagnosis, based on a heightened index of

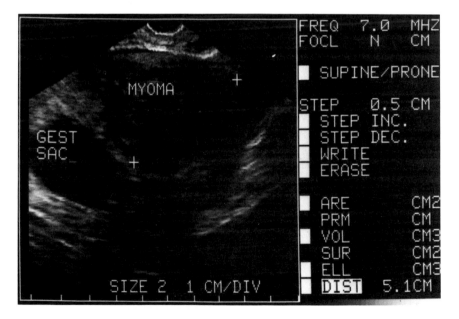

Fig. 7-7. This scan depicts a 5-cm lower uterine segment myoma. The most inferior portion of the gestational sac is also visualized. This patient had a history of repeated midtrimester pregnancy losses. Her myomatous uterus was not appreciated on clinical examination.

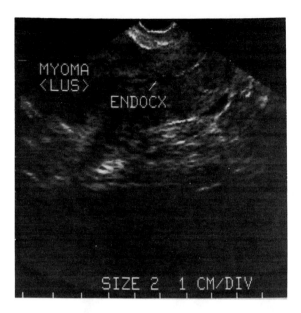

Fig. 7–8. This patient was preoperative for a cervical circlage procedure. She had a history of multiple midtrimester losses felt to be secondary to incompetent cervical os. Scan here depicts a normal thin linear sonolucent endocervical canal (ENDOCX). Multiple small lower uterine segment (LUS) myomas previously undiagnosed were noted. Thus an inappropriate circlage procedure was avoided after endovaginal ultrasound made the correct diagnosis.

suspicion and liberal use of tocolytic agents, is the cornerstone to improving outcome.

A reliable diagnosis of premature labor is sometimes difficult to make. If the physician waits until obvious cervical dilatation has taken place, then the likelihood of success with tocolytic agents may be diminished. By the same token, patients are often begun on tocolytic agents, and uterine contractility is still apparent on external fetal monitoring. Endovaginal ultrasound scanning techniques can image the endocervical canal and the area of the internal os (Fig. 7–9). Objective analysis of the state of the internal os and the presence or absence of "funneling" of the amniotic sac at the level of the internal os can be accurately diagnosed and followed with endovaginal ultrasound (Figs. 7–10, 7–11). The clinician, however, should be cautioned against overreliance on objective findings in making the initial decision to begin tocolytic agents or furthermore deciding when to discontinue them.

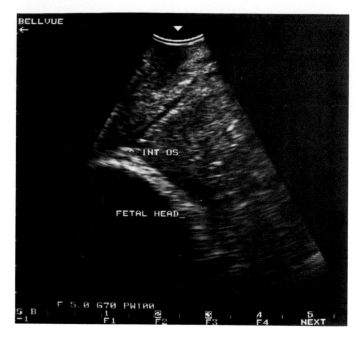

Fig. 7–9. Normal endocervical canal. The area of the internal os (INT OS) is easily recognized. Note the portion of fetal head overlying the cervix.

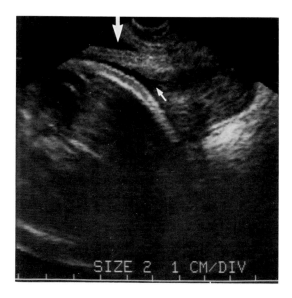

Fig. 7–10. Very slight funneling (small arrow) of the sac in the region of the endocervical canal. The fetal head is seen proximal to this. Also note very small amount of urine in the urinary bladder anteriorly (large arrow).

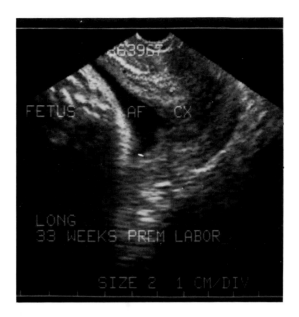

Fig. 7–11. Patient at 33 weeks gestation in clinically evident premature labor. Endovaginal scan here shows marked funneling of the amniotic sac overlying the region of the cervix (CX). AF, amniotic fluid.

LOWLYING PLACENTA/PLACENTA PREVIA

Not infrequently ultrasound scans performed in conjunction with amniocentesis procedures or for dating and fetal anatomical survey (between 18 and 22 weeks) may reveal the existence of "lowlying placenta, cannot rule out marginal previa." The so-called placental migration, which shows that the vast majority of such cases are clearly not placenta previa if rescanned into the third trimester, probably stems from the fact that the exact location of the placenta relative to the internal cervical os is difficult to assess accurately with traditional transabdominal ultrasound techniques. With endovaginal scanning techniques the cervix can be readily visualized; the endocervical canal will appear sonolucent and can be traced back to the internal os (Fig. 7–12). Whether placental tissue actually covers this structure can be discerned with the endovaginal approach (Fig. 7–13). Clinically such patients have a closed external cervical os and are not bleeding; even the most conservative of obstetricians/gynecologists would agree

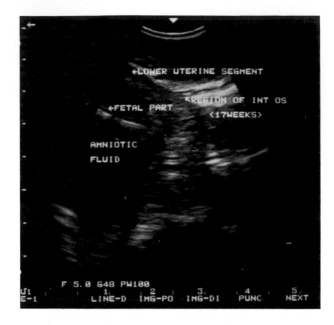

Fig. 7–12. Pregnancy at 17 weeks. The endocervical canal and region of the internal os (INT OS) are easily visualized as they enter the myometrium. A fetal part and the region of amniotic fluid are labeled.

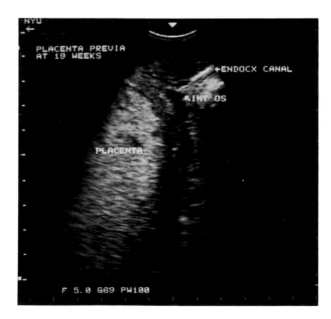

Fig. 7–13. Total placenta previa at 19 weeks. Placenta is seen here to overlie the region of the internal os (INT OS) going from anterior to posterior wall of the lower uterine segment. The relationship of the endocervical (ENDOCX) canal is clearly noted.

that placing a probe in the vaginal fornix in these patients at this time should produce no morbidity.

BLEEDING IN THE SECOND AND THIRD TRIMESTERS

Cases of overt bleeding in the second and third trimesters require a somewhat more conservative approach. Certainly abdominal ultrasound views can be obtained without a full urinary bladder to localize the general vicinity of the placenta. If placenta previa is definitively ruled out, then clinically one must consider the diagnosis of placental separation (abruption). In such a case, speculum exam followed by endovaginal ultrasound evaluation can and should be performed. Occasionally there will be causes of vaginal bleeding that may originate with the cervix itself (cervical laceration, cervical erosion, placental or endocervical polyp, or aborting myoma). If on speculum examination the cervix is closed and no obvious cervical source of bleeding is seen, then careful endovaginal ultrasound may be performed without ill effect. Remember that the ultrasound probe goes into the vaginal fornix and not the endocervical canal itself. Occasionally echoes that may be confusing even with an adequately filled urinary bladder using the transabdominal approach may be more easily interpreted with the endovaginal scanning technique. This may be especially true when attempting to distinguish fibroids from blood and blood clot in the lower uterine segment.

POSTPARTUM PERIOD

Endovaginal ultrasound can be helpful for some patients in the postpartum period. The postoperative cesarean section patient may have fever without an obvious source that may be accompanied by elevation of the white blood count and/or sedimentation rate as well as some nonspecific tenderness in the lower abdomen. Endovaginal ultrasound can easily identify any bladder flap hematoma when it is exists and can help to follow such collections objectively (Fig. 7-14). It should be noted, however, that even normal postoperative cesarean section patients without fever or symptoms may exhibit small sonolucent areas between the lower uterine segment and the bladder that obviously represent a small

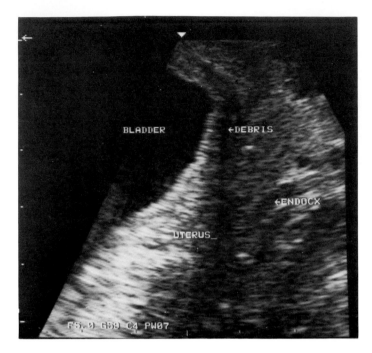

Fig. 7–14. Postoperative cesarean section patient with fever and elevated white blood cell count. Endovaginal scan revealed a collection of debris in the region of the bladder flap. This is a bladder flap hematoma, which resolved spontaneously with broad-spectrum antibiotic coverage.

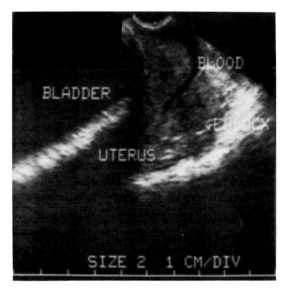

Fig. 7–15. Postoperative (day 3) cesarean section patient who was without symptoms. Note small sonolucency labeled blood in the region of the bladder flap. Such collections can be found almost routinely after low-flap cesarean section and are of no clinical significance.

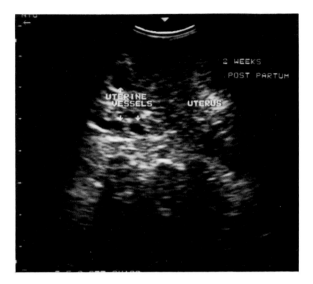

Fig. 7-16. Endovaginal scan 2 weeks postpartum after uncomplicated delivery and postpartum course. Prominent uterine vessels are seen lateral to the uterus. This is a normal finding and should not be confused for a pathological entity.

collection of blood and serum; such a collection should not always be considered abnormal (Fig. 7-15). Furthermore, on scanning patients in the postpartum period one should realize that the uterine vasculature, especially the dilate uterine veins, will be visualized, and they should not be mistaken for a pathological entity (Fig. 7-16).

SUGGESTED READINGS

Hansmann M, Hackeloer BJ, Staudock A. Ultrasound Diagnosis in Obstetrics and Gynecology. New York: Springer Verlag, 1985.

Jeanty P, Romero R. Obstetrical Ultrasound. New York: McGraw Hill, 1984.

Pritchard JA, MacDonald PC, Gant NF. Williams Obstetrics, Ed 17. Norwalk, CT: Appleton Century-Crafts, 1985.

Chapter 8

Ectopic Pregnancy

Ectopic pregnancy remains a major source of morbidity and even mortality in obstetrics and gynecology as we approach the end of the twentieth century. Before we can focus specifically on the role endovaginal ultrasound can play in ectopic pregnancy, we must first understand the different methods by which such patients come to our clinical attention.

THE "R/O ECTOPIC"

The "r/o ectopic" is a patient whose initial symptoms are even remotely suggestive of an ectopic pregnancy. There are varying degrees of our index of suspicion. Such a patient may be encountered in the clinic, in the office, in the emergency room, and occasionally even over the telephone. Astute clinicians, as they obtain historical information, are always asking themselves in the back of their minds—Is there any possible way that this patient could have an ectopic pregnancy? This is essential regardless of how atypical the presentation for ectopic is. Good history includes careful questioning about menses (remember, to many patients, all vaginal bleeding is a "period"), contraception, and any symptoms compatible with pregnancy (regardless of how subjective they seem). Obvious later symptoms (syncopy, shoulder pain, acute unilateral or lower abdominal pain, etc) can be asked about, but they are rarely present.

The first step is to include or exclude a pregnancy event. The method of choice would be a blood pregnancy hCG determination (a radioimmune assay specific for the beta-subunit of the hCG molecule). Barring a clinical lab error, there should be no false positives. Values can be quantitated and are reported in mIU/ml. The reader should be aware that there are two standards for reporting hCG levels. The International Reference Preparation (IRP) is the one employed by most early publications. The Second International Standard (2nd IS) are values that are approximately 50% of the IRP values. Increasingly more laboratories and publications are using hCG values reported in the 2nd IS rather than the IRP (see Chapter 4). It is essential for the reader to appreciate the difference between these two standards and to know which value their particular laboratory employs.

hCG is first detectable about 10 days after conception. Most qualitative tests are considered positive at hCG levels of 30 mIUs/ml (IRP), which is the level at the time of the expected menses (14 days postconception). In a normal IUG, the hCG level rises an average of 66% every 48 hours, or doubles about every 3 days. If the hCG level does not follow this pattern, all one can say is that this will not be a normal IUG—it may be an IUG destined to fail or it may be an ectopic pregnancy.

There are now more sensitive urinary tests that can be performed in 2 minutes. These are monoclonal antibody tests and are sensitive to hCG levels of 50 mIU/ml (IRP). Although blood hCG tests can be obtained from most labs in just a few hours, the ability to do a 2-minute test and get reliable qualitative results down to 50 mIU/ml (IRP) can be very useful clinically. It is also helpful to have a 2-minute urine slide agglutination test available. The sensitivities of these tests range from about 1,000 to 4,000 mIU/ml (IRP), depending on the manufacturer. Thus, if the monoclonal antibody test is negative, the patient is presumed not pregnant (hCG < 50 mIU/ml [IRP]). If the monoclonal antibody test is positive but the slide agglutination test is negative, the patient is indeed pregnant but the hCG level < 1,000 to 4,000 mIUml (IRP), depending on the test employed. If the slide agglutination test is positive, then of course the patient is pregnant, and the hCG level will be > 1,000–4,000 mIU/ml (IRP), depending on the test employed. So, by combining these two tests, you can get a semiquantitative assessment on a urine specimen in 2 minutes' time. This may be extremely valuable in interpreting ultrasound findings, as we will discuss below.

Once a pregnancy event has been documented, the clinician's index of suspicion may be raised by history of a previous ectopic, vaginal spotting, pain, or a palpable mass. The real value and main role of ultrasound in such cases lies in its ability to exclude the ectopic pregnancy by proving the presence of an IUG. For all practical purposes we discount the very rare possibility of coexisting intra- and extrauterine pregnancies (incidence in the range of 1 in 30,000 pregnancies). With more iatrogenic manipulation (in vitro fertilization, gamete intrafallopian transfer [GIFT] increasing ovulation induction), however, the actual incidence of this may be on the rise. Still it is felt the presence of an IUG indeed "rules out" an ectopic pregnancy.

At this point we must reintroduce the concept of the "discriminatory zone" of hCG. Originally described by Kadar et al. as 6,000–6,500 mIU/ml of hCG (IRP) and later modified by Nyberg et al. to 1,800 mIU/ml (2nd IS), it represents an attempt to find the level of hCG above which virtually all *normal* IUGs will visualize with ultrasound techniques. Preliminary work by this author and others indicates that the discriminatory zone of hCG with endovaginal ultrasound techniques is indeed much lower— in the range of 1,025 mIU/ml (IRP). This finding correlates with a maximal sac diameter of approximately 4 mm. Initial work also indicates that not only must the IUG be normal for early visualization, but also the uterus must be normal and homogenous in appearance. The presence of leiomyomata or coexisting IUDs (and the heterogenous echoes that such situations produce) may obscure the visualization of very early normal IUGs (see Chapter 4). Additionally, the endovaginal "discriminatory zone" may vary depending on the type and frequency of the equipment employed.

Keeping the above in mind, therefore, a normal IUG in a normal uterus should be recognizable with endovaginal ultrasound techniques if the hCG level exceeds 1,025 mIU/ml (IRP). There may indeed be other coexisting clinical findings to explain how the patient came to be a "rule out" ectopic. Such findings would include fluid in the cul-de-sac from a ruptured corpus luteum cyst, a coexisting corpus luteum cyst, an intrauterine pregnancy with evidence of subchorionic bleeding, and an intrauterine pregnancy that is definitely not normal (blighted ovum, missed abortion, or vanishing twin).

If the ultrasound is inconclusive (i.e., a definitive IUG is not visualized), then one must take serial hCG levels until an endovaginal scan would be conclusive. If an IUG is still not visualized, the appropriate next step in triage would be to perform a D&C. If the curettage material reveals chorionic villi, then one is dealing with an intrauterine pregnancy destined to failure. Villous mate-

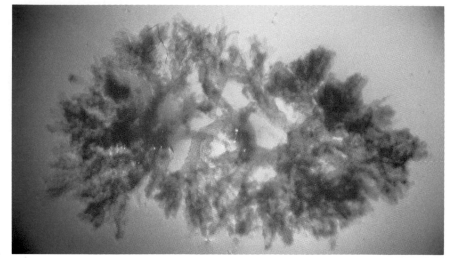

Fig. 8-1. (A) Entire placenta at 9 weeks LMP. Note secondary and tertiary budding and branching of the villi into chorion frondosum. Other primary villi attached to chorionic sac have regressed into chorion laeve (not pictured). **(B)** Secondary and tertiary villi (small arrow) and adjacent chorionic membrane on left (large arrow). When viewed under water these villi are lush and show "budding." While they do not actually "float," they do fall very slowly when suspended in water. With minimal training and experience they can be recognized when present with excellent reliability.

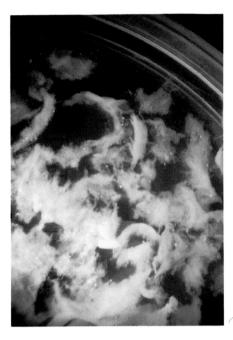

Fig. 8-2. Low-power magnification of maternal decidua, readily distinguished from villous material (placental in origin). Decidua will not display budding and branching as villi will. Decidual material will not suspend well and sinks rapidly to the bottom of a water-filled container.

rial (Fig. 8-1) may easily be differentiated from maternal decidua (Fig. 8-2) by "modified" (3×) low-power magnification of unstained curettage material. The widespread use of chorion villous sampling proves that with a small amount of training the clinician can easily distinguish villous material from decidual material. If no villous material is obtained at the time of curettage and if the patient has any history of vaginal bleeding, then follow-up hCG level must be obtained. A falling hCG level may be compatible with a diagnosis of complete abortion (occasionally tubal). The hCG level should be followed until it returns to 0. If the pregnancy is not in the uterus, as demonstrated by curettage, and if the hCG level rises subsequently, the findings are pathognomonic for an ectopic pregnancy, and definitive therapy can be carried out (Table 8-1).

TABLE 8-1. An Approach to the (R/O) Ectopic Pregnancy

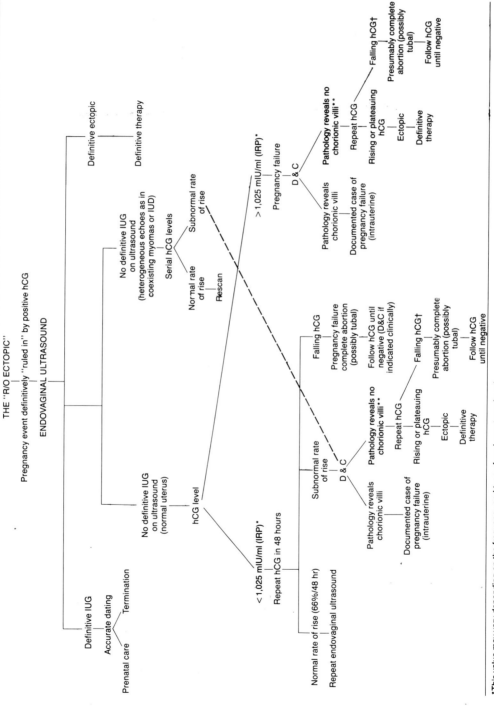

*This value may vary depending on the frequency and type of equipment employed.
**Assumes uterus has been completely emptied of tissue by D & C.
†Normal rate of fall of hCG with complete abortion is unknown.

UNSUSPECTED ECTOPIC PREGNANCY

The previous discussion centered on patients in whom there was a clinical suspicion of ectopic pregnancy. With the use of routine endovaginal ultrasound once pregnancy has been diagnosed, can unsuspected ectopic pregnancies be picked up before they manifest any signs or symptoms? Such patients can be divided into two categories—those wishing to continue and those wishing to terminate their pregnancies.

Those wishing to terminate their pregnancies can indeed benefit from routine pretermination ultrasound screening. As this subject is covered in Chapter 9, it will suffice to summarize here that pretermination ultrasound screening will: 1) pick up cases of unsuspected ectopic pregnancy; 2) reveal cases of unsuspected second-trimester pregnancies with inaccurate dates that can more safely be terminated by dilatation and evacuation (D&E) procedures; and 3) more accurately date pregnancies. Such absolute knowledge of gestational age can only serve to make the termination procedure that much safer.

Should patients presenting early in pregnancy with no suspicion of ectopic be routinely scanned in the first trimester at the time of their first exam? What the answer to this question will be in the future is unclear. Certainly concerns about bioeffects of endovaginal scanning techniques very early in pregnancy have not been studied exhaustively. Although intuitively felt to be safe, this remains to be proved. Obviously routine scanning would result in extremely accurate pregnancy dating. However, for patients early in the first trimester, concerns about dating can often be resolved nonsonographically. Furthermore, the resulting earlier diagnosis of all forms of pregnancy failure, including ectopics, may or may not outweigh the potential costs and theoretical bioeffects of such screening.

ULTRASOUND FINDINGS POTENTIALLY ASSOCIATED WITH ECTOPIC PREGNANCY

Appearance of the Endometrium

Endometrial findings in suspected ectopic pregnancies will include:

1. Normal IUG. As previously discussed, very early on one will see a gestational sac characterized by a trophoblastic

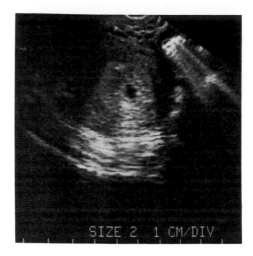

Fig. 8-3. Trophoblastic decidual reaction producing thick echogenic rind around a sonolucent center. This scan is 33 days LMP.

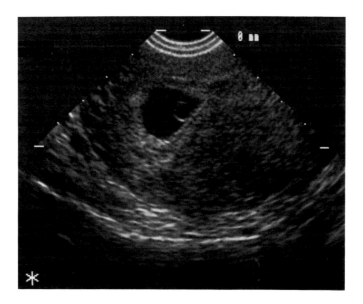

Fig. 8-4. The yolk sac is the first recognizable structure to develop normally within the early gestational sac. Previously some sonographers felt that the diagnosis of intrauterine pregnancy could not be absolutely made until a yolk sac had been demonstrated. Endovaginal scanning techniques, however, can reliably image an intrauterine pregnancy prior to the appearance of the yolk sac.

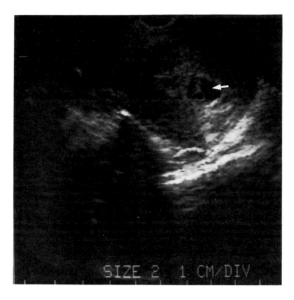

Fig. 8-5. A 6-mm embryonic pole (arrow), which demonstrated fetal cardiac activity, shown here lying adjacent to the extra-amniotic yolk sac.

decidual reaction. Sonographically it will be a thick echogenic rind around a sonolucent center (Fig. 8-3). Later one will see the yolk sac (Fig. 8-4) and finally an embryonic pole with fetal heart activity (Fig. 8-5).

2. Definitive IUG that may not be normal. As already discussed, this finding would include cases of subchorionic hemorrhage (Fig. 8-6) in the presence of fetal cardiac activity, pregnancy resorption (the blighted ovum [Fig. 8-7] or vanishing twin), or missed abortion.

3. Nondiagnostic endometrial findings. They may reveal decidual changes (sometimes previously called a decidual cast) or a "pseudosac," which could be compatible with ectopic pregnancy or intrauterine pregnancy not developing normally (Fig. 8-8A,B). There may be instances in which the endometrium has a secretory appearance (Fig. 8-9). *This finding does not exclude or make more likely the diagnosis of ectopic pregnancy.* Such cases need serial hCG levels and then either follow-up ultrasound scans or D&C as the next step in triage. Occasionally one may image a linear endometrial echo compatible with a complete abortion. Serial hCG levels still must be obtained to confirm such a diagnosis.

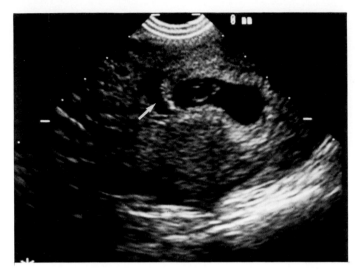

Fig. 8-6. Patient at 7.5 weeks LMP who had a positive pregnancy test and vaginal bleeding. Endovaginal scan performed for "r/o ectopic." IUG with fetal heart activity was noted. Sonolucent area outside the gestational sac represents subchorionic hemorrhage (arrow).

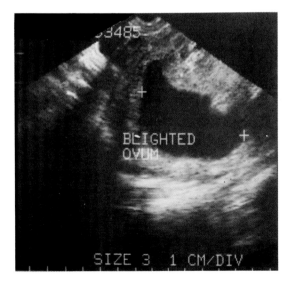

Fig. 8-7. Patient with positive pregnancy test, uncertain last menstrual period, clinically enlarged uterus, and history of vaginal bleeding. Endovaginal scan here reveals large irregular empty sac consistent with "blighted ovum."

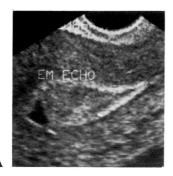

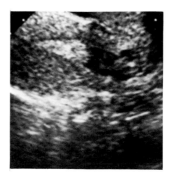

A   B

Fig. 8–8. (A) Endometrial (EM) echo highly magnified in patient with positive pregnancy test, vaginal bleeding, and abdominal pain. Such an endometrial echo is sometimes referred to as a "decidual cast" or "pseudogestational sac." In reality all one can definitively say is that this does not represent a normal gestational sac. There is no well-formed trophoblastic decidual reaction (see Fig. 8–3). **(B)** Endometrial echo, partially echogenic, contiguous with some area of blood and debris. Notice the similarity to **A.** Once again, all one can definitively say is that this is not a normal IUG. This patient ultimately revealed necrotic chorionic villi on D&C. Thus this was a case of early pregnancy failure, but still intrauterine. The patient in **A** had a leaking ectopic pregnancy.

EXTRAUTERINE FINDINGS

Adnexal Masses

Endovaginal ultrasound may reveal a coexisting intrauterine pregnancy and simple cystic adnexal mass (Fig. 8–10). Invariably this represents a corpus luteum cyst of the ovary. Occasionally coexisting with an intrauterine pregnancy there will be other adnexal pathologic conditions, such a hemorrhagic corpus luteum cyst, endometrioma, or possibly ovarian neoplastic process (whether benign or malignant).

Sometimes one will see an obvious extrauterine gestation, which may appear simply as a gestational sac with its typical echogenic rind around a sonolucent center (Fig. 8–11). Less frequently, but more reliably, one may see a yolk sac or even an embryonic pole with fetal cardiac activity within an extrauterine gestational sac (Fig. 8–12). Endovaginal ultrasound will be more successful at imaging such pregnancies than traditional transabdominal techniques. It is unclear exactly how often this will be true.

Visualization capability for an extrauterine pregnancy can be summarized as follows: the more normal in appearance a gesta-

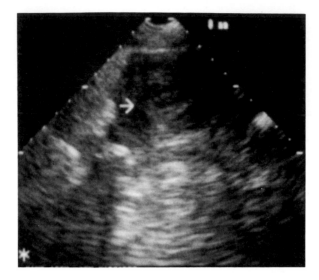

Fig. 8–9. Echogenic thick endometrial echo (arrow). Beta-subunit in this case was 394 mIU/ml (IRP). One can see such an appearance in the secretory or decidual stages of the nonpregnant patient. In addition, an ectopic pregnancy can yield an endometrium with this appearance. Once again, all one can definitively say is that this is not a normal intrauterine pregnancy. D&C on this patient revealed degenerating chorionic villi. Thus correct diagnosis was missed abortion.

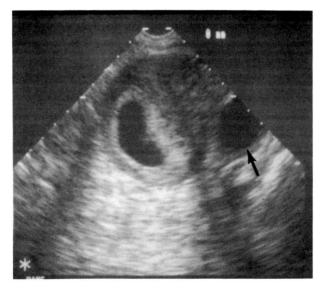

Fig. 8–10. Early intrauterine pregnancy with small coexisting corpus luteum cyst (arrow). Patient had a positive pregnancy test and right-side abdominal pain. Pelvic examination revealed slightly enlarged uterus and the presence of a right adnexal mass. Endovaginal ultrasound made the proper diagnosis.

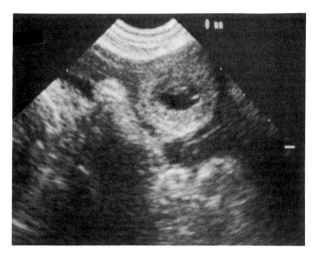

Fig. 8–11. Well-formed extrauterine gestation (highly magnified), appearing much like a normal gestational sac (i.e., echogenic rind around a sonolucent center), except that it was located outside the uterus. Remember that the more normal in appearance a gestation is (regardless of location inside or outside the uterus), the more likely it will be imaged with ultrasound.

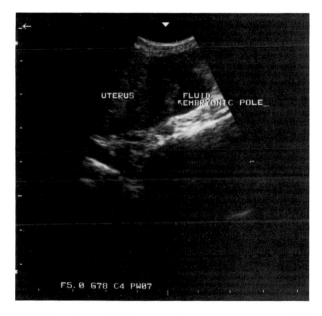

Fig. 8–12. A definitive diagnosis of extrauterine pregnancy was made here by imaging a 1-cm embryonic pole with fetal cardiac activity. It is seen lying outside and lateral to the uterus within some free fluid. Such a definitive diagnosis allows one to proceed directly to laparotomy.

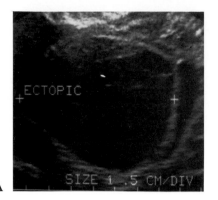 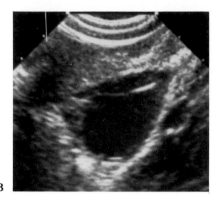

Fig. 8-13. **(A)** Highly magnified adnexal mass seen in the patient whose endometrium is imaged in Figure 8–8A. In spite of the labeling, such nondiagnostic findings in the adnexa do not necessarily represent a definitive extrauterine gestation. See Figure 8–13B for comparison. **(B)** Adnexal mass imaged in the patient in Figure 8–8B, representing a corpus luteum cyst with a small amount of debris within it from hemorrhage. This patient never had laparotomy secondary to pathological examination of D&C material revealing necrotic chorionic villi. The adnexal cystic mass had resolved at the time of the patient's 2-week follow-up examination.

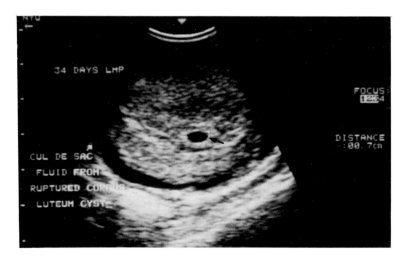

Fig. 8-14. Patient at 34 days LMP with acute onset of lower abdominal pain. Endovaginal scan revealed a 7-mm intrauterine pregnancy (black arrow) with fluid filling the cul-de-sac from a ruptured corpus luteum cyst.

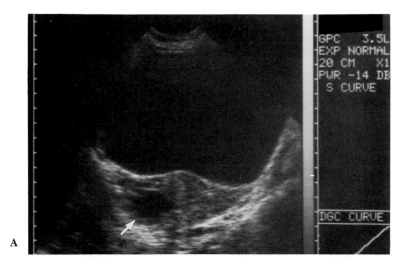

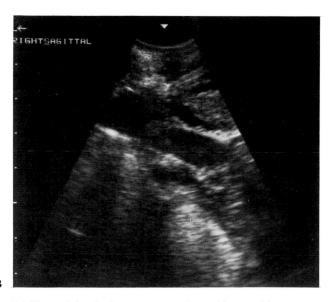

Fig. 8–15. (A) Transabdominal scan on a patient with a positive pregnancy test, no IUG seen within the uterus, and an ill-defined mostly sonolucent mass posterior and to the right of the uterus, which was felt to be a possible right-sided ectopic pregnancy (arrow). **(B)** Endovaginal scan of the right posterior aspect of the pelvis, representing loops of small bowel that showed no peristalsis during real-time examination. Endovaginal scan of the left side revealed an embryonic pole outside the uterus (see Fig. 8–12). At laparotomy several loops of small bowel were seen sitting in a small amount of free blood that resulted in a focal ileus. In endovaginal scanning, normal bowel will be seen throughout the pelvis. It is recognized by the motion that peristalsis produces. The sonographer must come to realize that a focal or total ileus will result in the bowel producing bizarre complex echoes that may often be confusing because of the lack of peristalsis.

tion is, regardless of whether it is located inside or outside the uterus, the more likely it is to be imaged with ultrasound techniques (whether endovaginal or transabdominal methods are employed). A *definitive* diagnosis of ectopic pregnancy on ultrasound requires at least a true sac and, better still, an embryonic pole. Not all adnexal masses, even when there is no IUG within the uterus, will be ectopic pregnancies. Cases of intrauterine pregnancy failure can have cystic adnexal masses (Fig. 8–13A,B). The clinician should be cautioned against "overcalling" definitive ectopics and should still consider D&C to look for chorionic villi in such cases.

Pelvic fluid can be easily imaged with endovaginal scanning techniques. Occasionally it will be seen with a coexisting intrauterine pregnancy, as in cases of ruptured corpus luteus cysts (Fig. 8–14). At other times pelvic fluid will represent the presence of hemoperitoneum. Occasionally there will be a focal paralytic ileus in the region of pelvic collections of blood. This can give off very confusing and diffuse echo patterns associated with bowel if peristalsis is not present (Fig. 8–15A,B).

SUMMARY

Endovaginal ultrasound will improve our handling of ectopic pregnancy by: 1) earlier diagnosis of IUG when present and when normal; 2) greater likelihood of definitively imaging an extrauterine pregnancy when present; and 3) bringing the imaging aspect of diagnosis back to the clinician in the office. The availability of endovaginal ultrasound in the practioner's office should cut down considerably on the frequency of having to refer the patient elsewhere for evaluation, thus this will save time. This will also save potential errors that are compounded each time one physician must convey clinical information to another physician. By reducing the number of people involved, we should see the best possible synthesis of all available clinical information.

SUGGESTED READINGS

Batzer FR, Weiner S, Corson SL, et al. Landmarks during the first forty-two days of gestation demonstrated by the β-sub-unit of human chorion gonadotropin and ultrasound. Am J Obstet Gynecol 146:973–979, 1983.

Bradley WG, Fiske CE, Filly RA. The double sac sign of early intrauterine pregnancy: Use in exclusion of ectopic pregnancy. Radiology 143:223–226, 1983.

Breen J. A 21-year survey of 654 ectopic pregnancies. Am J Obstet Gynecol 106:1004–1019, 1970.

Filly RA. Ectopic pregnancy: The role of sonography. Radiology 162:661–668, 1987.

Goldstein SR, et al. Subchorionic bleeding in threatened abortion: Sonographic findings and significance. Am J Roentgenol 141:975–978, 1983.

Goldstein SR, et al. Combined sonographic pathologic surveillance in elective first trimester terminations. Obstet Gynecol 71:747–750, 1988.

Goldstein SR, et al. Very early pregnancy detection with endovaginal ultrasound. Obstet Gynecol 72:200–204, 1988.

Kadar N, DeVore G, Romero R. Discriminatory hCG zone. Its use in sonographic evaluation for ectopic pregnancy. Obstet Gynecol 58:156–161, 1981.

Kadar N, Taylor KJW, Rosenfield AT. Combined use of serum hCG and sonography in the diagnosis of ectopic pregnancy. Am J Roentgenol 141:609–615, 1983.

Nyberg DA, Filly RA, Mahony BS, et al. Early gestation: Correlation of hCG levels and sonographic identification. Am J Roentgenol 144:951–954, 1985.

Nyberg DA, Filly RA, Duarte Filho DL, et al. Abnormal pregnancy: Early diagnosis by US and serum chorionic gonadotropin levels. Radiology 158:393–396, 1986.

Nyberg DA, Laing FC, Filly RA. Threatened abortion: Sonographic distinction of normal and abnormal gestation sacs. Radiology 158:397–400, 1986.

Reece EA, Petrie RH, Sirmans MF. Combined intrauterine and extrauterine gestations: A review. Am J Obstet Gynecol 146:323–330, 1983.

Romero R, Kadar N, Copel JA, et al. The effect of different human chorionic gonadotropin assay sensitivity on screening for ectopic pregnancy. Am J Obstet Gynecol 153:72–74, 1985.

Subramanyam BR, Raghavendra BN, Balthazar EJ, et al. Hematosalpinx in tubal pregnancy: Sonographic-pathologic correlation. Am J Roentgenol 141:361–365, 1983.

Weiner C. The pseudogestational sac in ectopic pregnancy. Am J Obstet Gynecol 139:959–961, 1981.

Weinstein L, Morris MB, Dotters D, Christian CD. Ectopic pregnancy—a new surgical epidemic. Obstet Gynecol 61:698–701, 1983.

Chapter 9

Routine Use of Ultrasound Prior to First-Trimester Termination

There are more than 1.3 million elective terminations of pregnancy performed annually in this country. Of these, 90% are first-trimester, and 50% are ≤ 8 weeks from the last menstrual period. Although only 10% of pregnancy terminations are performed in the second trimester, they account for 50% of the mortality associated with the procedure. In the past, routine ultrasound prior to elective termination of pregnancy was not recommended or performed. Some of the resistance was the feeling that such a procedure was not "cost-effective." This may indeed be true if the patient must be sent from the Ob-Gyn office to the radiologist for a "pelvic scan" prior to the scheduling and performance of the termination procedure.

DEMOGRAPHICS

For background, we must first discuss some of the demographics associated with the performance of pregnancy terminations. Among Ob-Gyn physicians, 42% perform terminations of pregnancy. Among family practitioners and general surgeons, 3% of each group perform such procedures. Of the total number of physicians performing such procedures, 3% account for 50% of the volume of pregnancy terminations. For these physicians, that is an average caseload of 35 per week.

Of first trimester terminations, 75% are done in free-standing clinics where there is a fairly large volume—enough to be prepared for the special considerations of the procedure, such as analgesia/anesthesia, blood typing, pathology concerns, and, in our opinion, ultrasonography. Approximately 25% of terminations are done in a hospital setting (usually in ambulatory surgery) or in physicians' offices. Obviously these patients would usually visit the doctor's office before scheduling such day surgery, and if ultrasound equipment is available in these doctors' offices, it could and should be used.

Pregnancy termination morbidity can be reduced if unsuspected ectopic pregnancies are identified at the time of termination and if precise dating information is available prior to the performance of the procedure. Precise dating could prevent inadvertent performance of second-trimester procedures, as well as allow for appropriate surgical dilatation. Overdilatation is a major factor in tears to the lower uterine segment.

SURVEILLANCE

We have developed a combined sonographic-pathological surveillance of elective first-trimester pregnancy terminations. Such a protocol was developed at a fairly large free-standing clinic in New York City, which does an average of 20–45 pregnancy termination a day. The protocol was developed before the advent of endovaginal ultrasound probes. Each patient with a positive pregnancy test is seen in an "ultrasound room" where a transabdominal "empty bladder" ultrasound is performed. We use the phrase empty bladder because the patients are kept—nothing by mouth (NPO)—for anesthesia considerations and are routinely asked to void upon arrival at the clinic to provide urine for a urinary pregnancy test. Thus their urinary bladders are empty out of necessity. If it was felt necessary, the urinary bladder could be filled by drinking water (which would render the patient no longer NPO and necessitate postponing the procedure) or by Foley catheter insertion and filling of the urinary bladder. Such a procedure does not lend itself to screening in an out-patient setting.

With this empty bladder technique, it is noteworthy that after 8 weeks LMP all gestational sacs are identified regardless of orientation of the uterus. We found that approximately 80% of patients had anteverted uteri and 20% retroverted. When the uterus is anteverted, 98% of all pregnancies with a positive routine urinary pregnancy test were visualized with an empty bladder transabdominal technique (Fig. 9-1). However, when the uterus was retroverted, only 57% of gestational sacs were visualized at 8 weeks LMP or less (Fig. 9-2). We found a 1.6% incidence (4 out of 250) of patients who by dates were in the first trimester but who sonographically were found to be actually in the second trimester (13, 14, 14, and 16 weeks). These patients were referred to hospital for dilatation and evacuation (D&E) procedures.

The termination procedures were then performed, and a "modified" gross examination of unstained curettage material using 3× magnification was carried out. It became obvious that tissue of placental origin (chorionic villi) (Fig. 9-3A–C) can easily be distinguished from tissue of maternal origin (decidua only) (Fig. 9-4A,B). All patients who had evidence of an intrauterine sac on ultrasound had confirmation of an intrauterine pregnancy by modified gross pathological examination. There were 1.6% of patients (4 out of 250) who had no identifiable intrauterine pregnancy on ultrasound and had "decidua only" on modified gross pathological examination. Because there was no history of vaginal bleeding since the last menstrual period, these four patients were referred to hospital, where laparoscopy/laparotomy was performed the same day, revealing unruptured ectopic pregnancies in all four.

ENDOVAGINAL TECHNIQUES

We have since incorporated endovaginal scanning into our clinic setting. Patients are still scanned initially with an empty bladder transabdominal technique. If an intrauterine gestation is seen, it is documented and measured. Patients at greater than 12 weeks gestational age are retriaged for appropriate D&E procedures. If no intrauterine gestation is noted, then an endovaginal scan is performed. We find this necessary in approximately 9% of cases. If a definitive extrauterine pregnancy (Fig. 9-5) is visualized (0.3%), then obviously the patient is sent directly to hospital for appropriate definitive therapy. If no intrauterine pregnancy is seen on endovaginal scan, then the patient is appropriately counseled, and either the procedure is carried out and the tissue

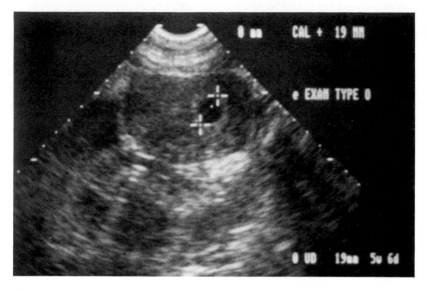

Fig. 9–1. Transabdominal "empty bladder" ultrasound of gestational sac (calipers) at 5.5 weeks LMP. Patient is NPO and has voided to give urine for pregnancy test, thus necessitating empty bladder. In some clinical settings, such empty bladder transabdominal scans will be a more efficient screening technique, thus reserving endovaginal scans for those cases in which no IUG is visualized.

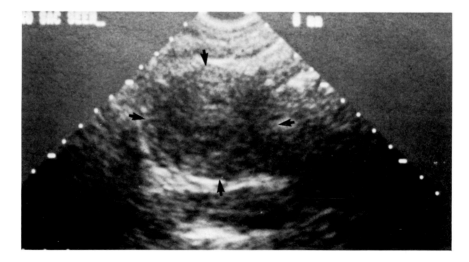

Fig. 9–2. "Empty bladder" transabdominal scan at 7 weeks LMP. Uterus (outlined by black arrows) was clinically retroverted at the time of termination. No sac was seen using this ultrasound technique, although a normal 7-week size gestation was recovered at the time of suction curettage and confirmed by modified gross pathological examination.

examined for evidence of chorionic villi, or a quantitative beta-subunit is obtained, and the patient is given potential ectopic precautions, with appropriate follow-up serial beta-hCG levels taken. We have previously demonstrated that with endovaginal scanning a normal intrauterine pregnancy can be visualized when the greatest sac diameter exceeds 4 mm and the beta-hCG level exceeds 1,025 mIU/ml (IRP) (see Chapter 4). It should be noted, however, that this will only be true of a *normal* pregnancy in a *normal* uterus. Uteri giving off heterogenous echoes (as in coexisting IUDs or multiple myomas) may make visualization of even normal very early pregnancies impossible. That is why even if one fails to visualize a pregnancy with beta-hCG levels greater than 1,025 mIU/ml (IRP), one should have the procedure performed and the tissue inspected for evidence of chorionic villi.

As noted in our clinic setting, it is more efficient timewise to begin with the transabdominal empty bladder ultrasound scan and reserve the endovaginal technique only for those cases in which the transabdominal technique is inadequate. It is only necessary for the patient to lower her pants to the region of the pubic symphysis in order to do a transabdominal scan. In our clinic, the endovaginal scan requires that the patient actually remove her garments, change into a gown, and be ready for essentially a pelvic examination. Obviously, for terminations performed in an office setting or when the physician schedules the procedure for a surgical unit, an in-office endovaginal ultrasound examination at the time of the physician's pelvic examination may be more efficient timewise.

A subsequent study of abortion surveillance with ultrasound was performed on 674 patients. All were ≤ 12 weeks from the last menstrual period. None had any history of vaginal bleeding. All had positive urinary pregnancy tests, although 28 had negative slide agglutination tests (sensitivity 4,000 mIU/ml (IRP) but positive monoclonal antibody tests (sensitivity 50 mIU/ml (IRP). All patients were initially scanned with a 3.5-MHz transducer using the empty bladder technique. The results showed that 91% demonstrated an intrauterine pregnancy on empty bladder transabdominal ultrasound. Of these, 17 cases (incidence 2.5%) were actually second-trimester cases with inaccurate menstrual histories. All of them were appropriately retriaged for D&E procedures.

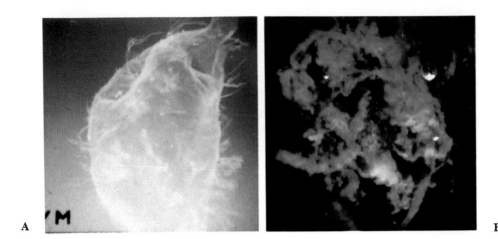

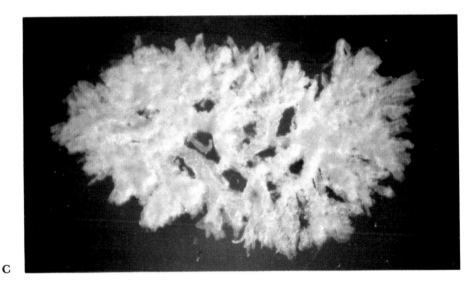

Fig. 9–3. **(A)** Chorionic sac (partially collapsed) at 5.5 weeks LMP. Note the primary villous projections attached to the chorionic sac. This early trophoblastic invasion into decidua results in the echogenic rind that produces the typical sonographic appearance of an early gestational sac. **(B)** Higher power magnification of chorionic villi at 9 weeks LMP. **(C)** Entire placenta at 8 weeks LMP. The chorionic sac is not visualized here. The chorionic villi have undergone branching and budding into secondary and tertiary villi known as chorion frondosum. Other portions of primary chorionic villi have regressed and are known as chorion laeve (not pictured).

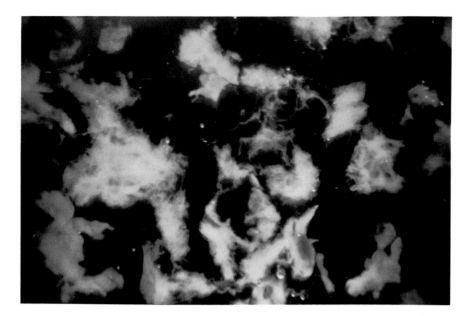

A

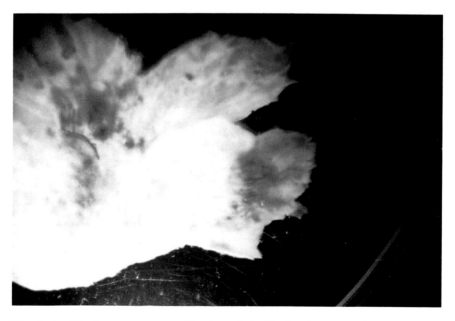

B

Fig. 9-4. (A) Low-power magnification of decidualized endometrial tissue. This material is totally of maternal origin. Thus the finding of such tissue alone at the time of termination, even if fairly large in volume, does not confirm the presence of an intrauterine pregnancy. **(B)** Higher power magnification of maternal decidua. This tissue lacks the finger-like projections of chorionic villi (see Fig. 9-3B for comparison).

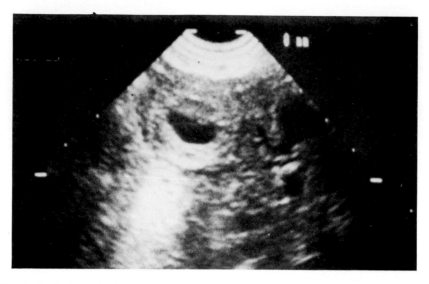

Fig. 9-5. Endovaginal scan revealing definitive gestational sac with an embryonic pole within it. The uterus is not seen in this scanning plane. This was an obvious definitive extrauterine pregnancy The patient was sent directly to hospital for appropriate exploratory laparotomy.

Nine percent (62 patients) required endovaginal ultrasound scans. Of these, 34 revealed an intrauterine gestation that was then confirmed at time of suction curettage and subsequent modified gross pathological examination. As previously stated, there were two unruptured ectopics definitively diagnosed by endovaginal ultrasound who were sent to hospital for definitive therapy. Of 21 remaining patients in whom no sac was seen on endovaginal ultrasound, D&C revealed chorionic villi on modified gross pathological exam in 17. The remaining four had pathological results that revealed "decidua only." Serial hCG levels in these patients revealed two ectopic pregnancies and two complete abortions (presumably tubal, since there was no history of any vaginal bleeding).

There is another aspect to the value of pretermination ultrasound screening. In our study we only addressed those patients felt to be in the first trimester by menstrual history who actually were in the second trimester. Such patients, if unrecognized, represent potentially high risk for serious morbidity and possibly even mortality. However, there will be patients in whom the gestational age will be significantly altered (either raised or low-ered) by ultrasound screening. For example, the patient who appears to be at 7 weeks gestational age by dates, and perhaps is difficult to examine because of obesity or an inability to relax, but in reality is at 11 weeks gestational age, may present a higher risk situation to the operator. Conversely, a patient who appears to be at 11 weeks gestational age by dates (and who is difficult to examine, possibly because of previous surgery, inability to relax, or presence of coexisting myoma) but in reality is only 7 weeks pregnant may find herself being unnecessarily overdilated. Over-dilatation is a major source of splitting of the endocervical canal and can lead to a tear into the descending branch of the uterine artery, resulting in hemorrhage and possible surgical intervention. In summary, absolute knowledge of gestational age prior to com-mencement of the termination procedure can only make the pro-cedure that much safer. There is wide variety in menstrual history and still, unfortunately, wide variety in clinical assessment of the uterine size. The use of ultrasound can help to bridge that gap.

Thus ultrasound screening prior to elective termination can identify unsuspected ectopic pregnancy at the time of termination. Such surveillance can also provide precise dating information prior to the procedure that will prevent inadvertent second-trimes-ter procedures from being performed and allow for appropriate cervical dilatation. Furthermore, whether to begin such screening transabdominally with endovaginal backup when indicated or begin primarily with the endovaginal technique will depend on where the procedure is being performed.

SUGGESTED READINGS

Abortion Surveillance. MMWR CDC Surveill Summ 32:1SS–7SS, 1983.

Centers for Disease Control. Ectopic Pregnancy Surveillance, 1970–1978. US Dept. of Health and Human Services. July, 1982.

Goldstein SR, Snyder JR, Watson C. The non-filled bladder: Special applications in the sonographic evaluation of the first trimester pregnancy prior to elective termination. J Bellevue Obstet Gynecol Soc 4:23–26, 1988.

Goldstein SR, et al. Combined sonographic pathologic surveillance in elective first trimester terminations. Obstet Gynecol 71:747–750, 1988.

Goldstein SR, et al. Very early pregnancy detection with endovaginal ultrasound. Obstet Gynecol 72:200–204, 1988.

Grimes D. Second trimester abortion in the United States. Fam Plann Perspect 16:260–266, 1984.

Kadar N, Caldwell BV, Romero R. A method of screening for ectopic pregnancy and its indications. Obstet Gynecol 58:162–166, 1981.

Kadar N, DeVore G, Romero R. Discriminatory hCG: Its use in the sonographic evaluation for ectopic pregnancy. Obstet Gynecol 58:156–161, 1981.

New York Codes, Rules and Regulations. Volume C, Chapter V, Section 751.9, 1985.

Nyberg D, Filly R, Filho D, et al. Abnormal pregnancy: Early diagnosis by ultrasound and serum chorionic gonadotropin levels. Radiology 158:393–396, 1986.

Chapter 10

Ovulation Induction
and Follicle Surveillance

Infertility affects approximately one out of every six couples in the United States. The postponement of initiation of childbirth by modern women until later stages of their reproductive life, in addition to the widespread prevalence of sexually transmitted pelvic infections, accounts for the dramatic increase in the numbers of infertile couples over the last 2 decades. It is calculated that of all couples experiencing reproductive difficulties, 30–40% of them will be identified as having absent or defective ovulation. Hypothalamic dysfunction and chronic anovulation syndromes with increased androgens (i.e., polycystic ovaries) are responsible for the majority of these cases.

With the development of effective pharmacological agents for induction of ovulation, anovulatory infertility is at the present time being managed with great success. Pregnancy rates obtained with medical therapy when anovulation is the sole etiological factor of infertility are very rewarding.

Induction of ovulation has gained in sophistication over the past years and has therefore created the necessity for a reliable method of accurate monitoring. Careful monitoring of stimulated cycles is important to prevent complications from hyperstimulation and to optimize the chances of pregnancy by predicting when ovulation will occur. Timing of ovulation is also useful when timed intervention is required and can be done with great precision. The introduction of in vitro fertilization (IVF) for the treat-

This chapter was prepared by Benjamin Sandler, M.D., and Lawrence Grunfeld, M.D.

ment of a wide spectrum of infertility disorders requires "controlled hyperstimulation" in order to increase the number of oocytes available for fertilization.

PHARMACOLOGY OF OVULATION INDUCTION

Clomiphene citrate (CC) is a nonsteroidal agent, distally related to diethylstilbestrol (DES). Its similarity to the structure of C_{18} (estrogen) compounds is the basis of its mechanism of action, binding to hypothalamic estrogen receptors that subsequently activate the neuroendocrine mechanism for follicle-stimulating hormone (FSH) and luteinizing hormone (LH) production. FSH and LH, in turn, stimulate follicular growth. CC is regarded as the first line of treatment in patients with anovulation. The starting dose is 50 mg/day × 5 days, beginning on the fifth day of the cycle. Since the multiple pregnancy rate is only about 5% and severe hyperstimulation is almost nonexistent, intense ultrasound and hormonal surveillance is not necessary. When ultrasound scans of clomiphene citrate-stimulated cycles are performed, follicles are noted to be slightly larger (1–2 mm) than menotropinstimulated follicles (Fig. 10–1).

Human menopausal gonadotropins (HMG) are available for clinical use as a combination of FSH and LH (Pergonal) and as a preparation of pure FSH (Metrodin). Since they are powerful ovulation induction agents, menotropin-stimulated patients demand close surveillance during the treatment cycle. Serial ultrasound examinations and daily E_2 determinations in the preovulatory phase are mandatory. We routinely perform the first vaginal sonogram after 5 or 6 days of Pergonal stimulation (cycle day 8). When follicles reach maturity, determined by both follicular diameters and hormonal levels, human chorionic gonadotropin (hCG), 5,000–10,000 units, is given in order to trigger ovulation. The dose of HMG is tailored on an individual basis according to the patient's response. The multiple pregnancy rate is estimated to reach 20–25%.

Hyperstimulation syndrome is the most feared complication of menotropin use and occurs in its mild form in approximately 20% of all cycles and over 50% of conception cycles. Only 1–2% of patients will need to be hospitalized for severe overstimulation. The syndrome is characterized by increased capillary permeability, with consequent fluid shifts, hemoconcentration, and decreased renal perfusion (Fig. 10–2). Selection, recruitment, and

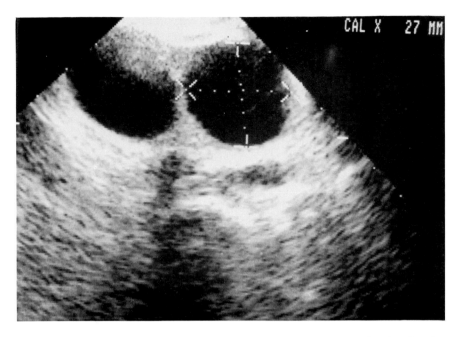

Fig. 10-1. Preovulatory vaginal ultrasound in a clomiphene citrate-stimulated cycle.

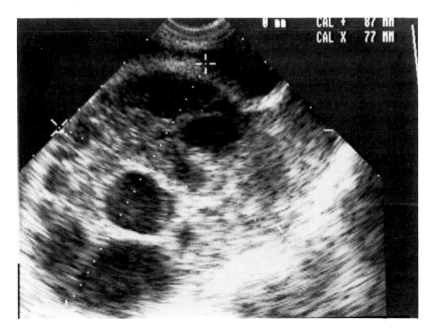

Fig. 10-2. Hyperstimulation syndrome with an enlarged ovary measuring 8.7 cm × 7.7 cm.

stimulation of multiple maturing oocytes is characteristic of Pergonal stimulation. Size determinations of each of the sonographically significant (> 10 mm in diameter) follicles should be obtained daily (Fig. 10–3). Occasionally, hCG is withheld after a large number of follicles are matured, in order to reduce the possibility of multiple pregnancy and hyperstimulation.

ULTRASOUND AND FOLLICULAR SURVEILLANCE

Since the advent of real-time sonography, ultrasound has been widely recognized as a valuable technique in assessing follicular development, growth, and timing of ovulation. Serial ultrasonographic determinations of follicular size would also provide clinicians with the necessary information to assess individual reponse to the induction therapy. For timed procedures like oocyte aspiration in the preovulatory stage for in vitro fertilization or timed artificial inseminations, monitoring follicular development is imperative.

Prior to the establishment of high-resolution real-time sonography for ovarian and follicular imaging in the mid-1970s, monitoring of stimulated cycles utilized hormonal (i.e., estradiol—E_2) determinations by radioimmunoassay. Other clinical parameters used to predict or establish ovulation include lower genital tract changes (i.e., cervical mucus) and basal body temperature graphics, both of which lack accuracy and consistency.

Multiple studies have compared the efficacy of serial ultrasound follicular size determinations against endocrinological parameters. It has been demonstrated that a linear correlation exists between the follicular diameters and the level of plasma estradiol during the preovulatory phase, since at 5–6 days prior to ovulation, the growth of the dominant follicle during the proliferative phase is constant at a rate of 1.5–2 mm per day until follicular rupture and excursion of the oocyte actually occurs (Fig. 10–4).

In the normal, nonstimulated cycle, 90% of the peripheral estradiol level arises from the dominant follicle. When pharmacologic agents for ovulation induction are used, the expected linear relation between E_2 and follicular diameters might not exist. During stimulated cycles, peripheral E_2 values are dependent on the number of recruited ovum. Frequently preovulatory oocytes are found at different maturational stages, each of them contributing to the total estrogen pool.

Ultrasound and serial estrogen determinations have a complementary role in follicle surveillance. Follicle size appears to corre-

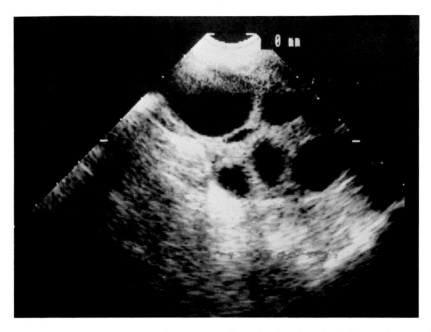

Fig. 10–3. Human menopausal gonadotropin, stimulated cycle with recruitment of multiple follicles at different maturational stages.

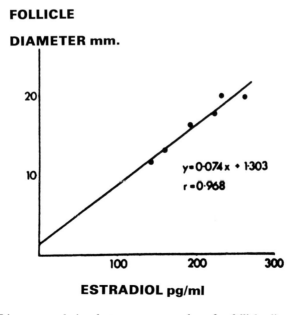

Fig. 10–4. Linear correlation between mean values for follicle diameter and mean levels of estradiol (E_2) on day −5 to day 0. (Reproduced from Hackeloer et al., 1979, by permission of the publisher.)

late reliably with maturity of the oocyte. When their largest diameter measures between 16 mm and 24 mm, the oocyte will be mature, and the follicle will have a normal complement of granulosa cells.

NORMAL CYCLE

During the normal menstrual cycle, endovaginal ultrasound is able to recognize follicular as well as endometrial changes. The dominant follicle that eventually will rupture is selected from a cohort of follicles in which the lesser ones are destined to become atretic. The initiation of follicular growth is a continuous process independent of gonadotropin stimulation that requires FSH and LH priming for its final development. Under proper stimulation, follicles that reach a minimal diameter of 14 mm will harbor a mature oocyte. Ovulation is not detected and pregnancies are not produced when the leading follicle does not reach at least 14 mm. Once the leading Graafian follicle reaches this point, the daily growth rate is approximately 1.5–2 mm in diameter until the time of ovulation, which usually occurs when the largest diameter reaches 20–24 mm (Fig. 10–5). Subordinate small follicles do not contribute significantly to the pool of estrogens. Therefore estradiol determinations correlate well with follicle measurements in the natural cycle.

The dominant follicle is clearly identified approximately 1 week prior to ovulation and can be followed with serial ultrasound until ovulation is demonstrated. The rapidly increasing amount of estrogens produced has a positive role for the establishment of the LH surge, with consequent luteinization of the granulosa cells. The LH surge is a reliable sign of impending ovulation and a necessary stimulus for follicular rupture. Ovulation will take place 34–36 hours after the initiation of the surge, and at 1–14 hours after its peak. While LH is being produced, progesterone is initially secreted by the luteal cells, in increasing amounts until the midsecretory phase of the cycle (Fig. 10–6).

Characteristic sonographic events at the time of ovulation have been portrayed, and actual follicular rupture has even been observed. Changes include diminution in follicular size, blurring of the borders, appearance of intrafollicular echoes (corpus hemorrhagicum) and demonstration of free fluid in the cul-de-sac. Thereafter, an irregular, mildly echogenic cystic structure repre-

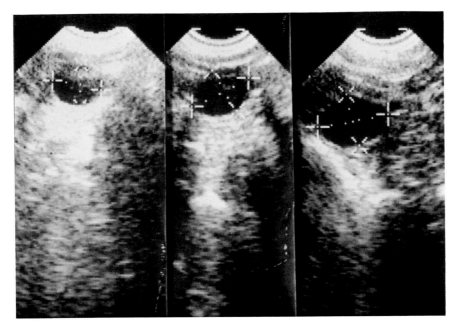

Fig. 10–5. Serial endovaginal scan demonstrating growth of leading preovulatory follicle in the normal cycle. Days 12, 13, 14.

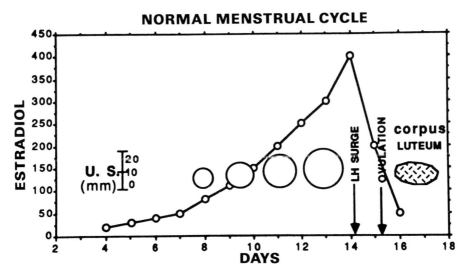

Fig. 10–6. Sequence of events in a nonstimulated cycle.

senting the corpus luteum diminishes in size throughout the secretory phase of the cycle until final luteolysis preceeding menses (Fig. 10–7).

The endometrium, as a hormonal-dependent tissue, demonstrates marked changes throughout the menstrual cycle. From a thin echo line during the proliferative phase, the endometrial stripe becomes thicker as the cycle advances as a function of glandular and stromal hyperplasia. A sonolucent halo around the more echogenic endometrial canal represents stromal edema. Throughout the luteal phase, the endometrial stripe regresses unless pregnancy occurs.

ADVANTAGES OF ENDOVAGINAL ULTRASOUND

Since the implementation of vaginal transducers in high-resolution, real-time ultrasound scanners, endovaginal ultrasound is now the preferred scanning method. Because of the proximity of

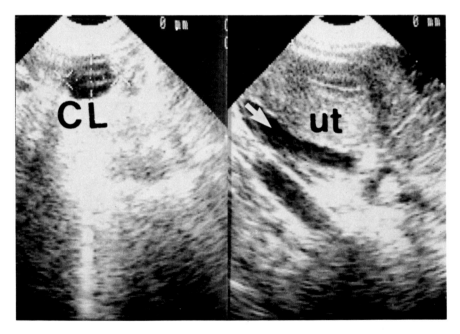

Fig. 10–7. Ultrasonographic postovulatory changes. On the left, a mildly echogenic corpus luteum. On the right, the arrow is pointing at fluid in the posterior cul-de-sac.

the pelvic organs to the vaginal fornices and, therefore, the tip of the vaginal probe, this new modality offers improved resolution in the identification of the pelvic structures. Since almost always the ovary is located within 4 cm of the scanning probe, great anatomical detail is obtained. During stimulation cycles, the ovaries enlarge and fill the posterior cul-de-sac or pouch of Douglas. The vaginal approach is advantageous to scan follicules and to perform aspiration procedures for oocyte retrieval in in vitro fertilization/embryo transfer (IVF/ET) programs.

One of the greatest advantages of endovaginal ultrasound relates to the fact that an overdistended bladder is not required as an "acoustic window." This immediately translates into elimination of patient discomfort due to a full bladder, especially in busy ultrasound units where patients may have to wait for scanning.

Patients with severe intrapelvic adhesions and obese patients may not be well visualized with abdominal techniques because of marked tissue attenuation. Adequate follicular delineation is in some cases practically impossible. Some studies recently published have compared the efficacy of follicular monitoring of both endovaginal and abdominal modes. As far as follicle size determination is concerned, both methods are acceptable, as long as the abdominal examination is optimal. Some investigators have compared both techniques in stimulated patients receiving a combination of clomiphene citrate and human menopausal gonadotropins. In women with a difficult or suboptimal examination secondary to obesity or severe pelvic adhesive disease, imaging improvement can be obtained in patients who are scanned vaginally (Fig. 10–8A and B). Endovaginal probes are ideal not only for follicular surveillance but also for visualization of the endometrial changes.

Excellent delineation and morphological detail is obtained, not only with large follicles but also when smaller cysts are present. Intrafollicular structures like the cumulus oophorus can be visualized in nearly one-third of all preovulatory follicles.

SCANNING TECHNIQUE

With the patient in semilithotomy position, the uterus is first localized in the midline and used as a reference point. Both longitudinal or sagittal and transverse or coronal views should be obtained to determine uterine size, shape, and position. The

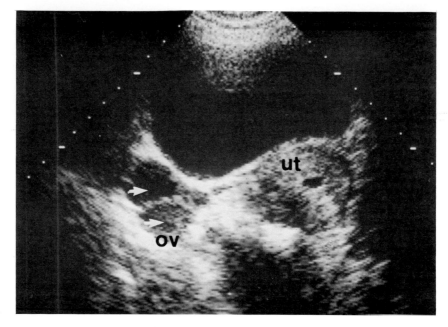

A

B

Fig. 10–8. Comparison of abdominal (**A**; arrows pointing at two follicles) and vaginal (**B**) ultrasound in an obese patient. Note improved resolution using endovaginal ultrasound technique. Abdominal mode is hampered by tissue attenuation.

ovaries are subsequently localized by directing the transducer at the lateral fornices. During stimulated cycles the ovaries are easily found, mainly through the presence of multiple echo-free cystic structures that represent growing follicles. The ovarian stroma has a characteristic uniform acoustic density similar to the myometrial tissue echogenicity.

Different methods for follicular measurements are used. Since follicles are not perfectly spherical, measurement of 3 diameters will allow us to calculate intrafollicular volume by using the formula $\pi/6 \times A \times B \times C$, where A, B, and C are diameters measured in three different planes. Volume calculations have been shown to correlate very accurately with the amount of fluid aspirated at the time of egg harvesting. For practical purposes, nevertheless, we routinely obtain two measurements: the largest diameter measured from the outer edge of the cyst wall to the opposite inner edge, and a perpendicular diameter. The calculated mean is used to estimate maturity status. In menotropin-stimulated cycles, follicles with a mean diameter of 16–18 mm have

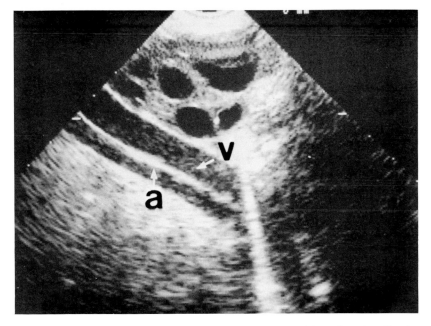

Fig. 10–9. Longitudinal view of a stimulated right ovary with perfect visualization of iliac artery (a) and vein (v) (medial).

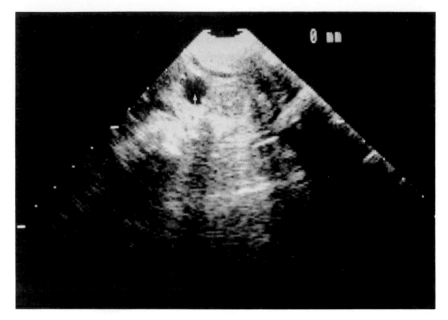

A

B

Fig. 10–10. Hydrosalpinx in cross section resembling a follicle (arrow) **(A)** and longitudinal view after rotating the transducer **(B)** shows typical sausage-shaped sonolucent appearance of a hydrosalpinx (arrow).

fully completed the maturational process and should yield fertilizable oocytes.

Follicles can sometimes be confused with other intrapelvic structures, mainly large-caliber blood vessels like the internal iliac artery and vein. They are differentiated by rotating the transducer 90° into a perpendicular plane. If the structure is a vessel, it will elongate on the screen and appear tubular (Fig. 10–9). Recognition of the hypogastric artery is obvious by its pulsations. Similarly, a hydrosalpinx or dilated fallopian tube can sometimes be confused with a follicle if seen in a cross-sectional plane (Fig. 10–10). Bowel has a relatively increased echogenicity and continued peristaltic movements that make discrimination easy for experienced sonographers.

SUMMARY

Ultrasonography is mandatory for the proper management of ovulation induction. Assessment of follicular maturity requires determination of the number and size of the developing follicles. Vaginal sonography offers several advantages over abdominal sonography, including improved resolution, easier identification of pelvic structures, and greater patient comfort. The combination of endocrinological and ultrasound measurements of follicular size will yield a safe and more successful therapy.

SUGGESTED READINGS

DeCherney AH, Laufer N. The monitoring of ovulation induction using ultrasound and estrogen. Clin Obstet Gynecol 27:4, 1984.

DeCrespingy L, O'Herling C, Robinson II. Ultrasonic observation of mechanism of human ovulation. Am J Obstet Gynecol 139:6, 1981.

Hackeloer B, Fleming R, Robinson H, et al. Correlation of ultrasonic and endocrinologic assessment of human follicular development. Am J Obstet Gynecol 135:1, 1979.

Kase N. Induction of ovulation. In Kase N, Weingold, (ed): Principles and Practice of Clinical Gynecology. New York: John Wiley and Sons, 1983.

Marrs R, Vargyas D, March C. Correlation of ultrasonic and endocrinologic measurements in human menopausal gonadotropin therapy. Am J Obstet Gynecol 145:4, 1983.

Meldrum D, Chetkowski R, Steingold K, et al. Transvaginal ultrasound scanning of ovarian follicles. Fertil Steril 42:5, 1984.

Nitschke-Dabelstein S. Monitoring of follicular development using ultrasonography. In Insler, Lunenfeld (eds): Infertility, Male and Female. Edinburgh: Churchill Livingstone, 1986.

Ritchie W. Ultrasound evaluation of normal and induced ovulation. Fertil Steril 43:2, 1985.

Schwimer S, Lebovic J. Transvaginal pelvic ultrasonography accuracy in follicle and cyst size determination. J Ultrasound Med 4:61, 1985.

Vargyas J, Marrs R, Kletzky O, Rushell D. Correlation of ultrasonic measurement of ovarian follicle size and serum estradiol levels in ovulatory patients following clomiphene citrate for in vitro fertilization. Am J Obstet Gynecol 144:5, 1982.

Yee B, Barnes R, Vargyas J, Marrs R. Correlation of transabdominal and transvaginal ultrasound measurements of follicle size and number with laparoscopic findings for in vitro fertilization. Fertil Steril 47:5, 1987.

Chapter 11

In Vitro Fertilization and Embryo Transfer

Surgical repair has been the only treatment available for damaged Fallopian tubes over the past 100 years. Although surgery is still preferred for the correction of ligated tubes, as well as for the treatment of endometriosis and some cases of pelvic adhesions, correction of tubal damage is not always possible. Surgery is not appropriate when the Fallopian tubes are absent or irreparably damaged. Furthermore, once surgical correction has been attempted, repeat surgery is usually associated with poor success. The poor results seen in severely damaged Fallopian tubes has led to a search for a Fallopian tube substitute. Animal experiments in which attempts to substitute other body organs, such as the ileum or carotid artery, or a plastic prosthesis to create a new Fallopian tube have met with failure. In humans, the Estes procedure, in which the ovary is transplanted directly into the endometrial cavity, was similarly unsuccessful in achieving pregnancies.

It was not until a decade ago that human in vitro fertilization (IVF) became an acceptable treatment for patients with uncorrectable tubal obstruction. As IVF evolved and became more commonly available, its indications widened. Currently IVF is performed to treat disorders such as unexplained infertility, immunological infertility, male factor infertility, and endometriosis. In fact, any infertility disorder can be treated with IVF, as long as there is a normal uterine cavity, a source of oocytes, and enough

This chapter was prepared by Lawrence Grunfeld, M.D., and Benjamin Sandler, M.D.

sperm to achieve fertilization. Advancements in ultrasound technology that have decreased the invasiveness of oocyte retrieval occurred simultaneously with IVF's proliferation and have made this procedure more acceptable for a wider range of infertility disorder.

Indications for IVF

Tubal obstruction

Endometriosis

Male factor

Immunologic

Unexplained

STEPS IN IN VITRO FERTILIZATION AND EMBRYO TRANSFER

Superovulation

Early in the course of in vitro fertilization's development it became apparent that the process of fertilizing an embryo and transferring it into the endometrial cavity is highly inefficient. Steptoe and Edwards first transferred single embryos that were recovered in natural cycles in 1977 and were able to achieve a 5% pregnancy rate. Although this was clearly a milestone in the advancement of therapy for infertility, early success rates would not be acceptable today. The major advancement resulting in an enhanced success was the use of hyperstimulation for the recruitment of many oocytes. Today, superovulation with human menopausal gonadotropins (HMG), and in some programs clomiphene citrate, is standard. Superovulation permits the retrieval of many oocytes, while in natural cycles only one oocyte matures. This increase in the pool of fertilizable oocytes will increase the number of embryos transferred into the endometrial cavity with a resultant increase in the chance of at least one embryo implanting.

In order to properly monitor hyperstimulated cycles, a combination of serum steroid measurements and ultrasound identification of follicles is utilized. While in normal cycles the level of serum estradiol parallels the growth of the single dominant follicle, in stimulated cycles this is not true. There is considerable asynchrony of follicular growth with the recruitment of follicles of various sizes. As not every follicle is similar in size, the contribution of each follicle to the circulating estradiol pool will differ. Serum estradiol, which is a product of the secretion of all developing follicles, cannot differentiate between a single large and several small follicles. Ultrasonography is, therefore, necessary to accurately assess the contribution of each follicle into the peripherally measured circulating estradiol pool.

Follicle Assessment

Asynchronous follicular growth characteristic of menotropin treatment is a result of early follicular development that occurs independently of gonadotropin stimulation. Follicles undergo a certain level of follicular growth and atresia even when gonadotropins are absent. When menotropins are initiated, follicles that have undergone some level of maturation will be stimulated. These follicles will be at different maturational stages and will be stimulated at a variable rate. This is in contrast to the natural cycle, in which only one follicle reaches maturity as gonadotropins steadily decline prior to ovulation. Ultrasound examination of the ovary in stimulated cycles demonstrates a variety of follicular sizes (Fig. 11–1).

Precise measurement of follicular diameters is vital to successful ovulation induction for IVF. In natural cycles, ovulation occurs at follicular diameters of 1.5–2.5 cm. Menotropin treatment, however, is associated with more rapid increases in oocyte maturity, as reflected by follicular diameters. Since only follicles that have achieved this level of stimulation will contain mature oocytes, it is important that oocyte aspiration be delayed until evidence of follicular maturation exists. Unlike ovulation induction in anovulatory women, it is the goal of in vitro fertilization to continue stimulation until all potential oocytes have matured, so that the maximum number of fertilizable oocytes can be retrieved. Consequently, it is not appropriate to trigger ovulation until most of the follicles have achieved a diameter of at least 1.5 cm.

While the mature (1.5–2.5 cm) follicles contain the fertilizable oocytes, the intermediate (1.0–1.5 cm) follicles also contribute to the hormonal production of the ovary. The goal of ovulation induction is the production of mature follicles containing fertilizable oocytes. The intermediate follicles are also important, how-

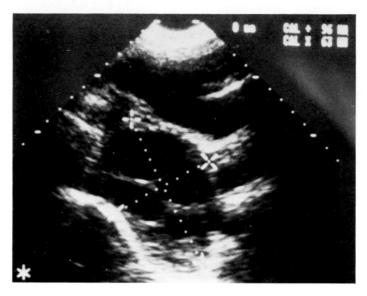

Fig. 11-1. Endovaginal view of stimulated ovary (in dotted cross) demonstrating follicular asynchrony. Note that all follicles are maximally demonstrated and vary in size.

ever, and may be responsbile for hyperstimulation, which can complicate ovulation induction. Abdominal sonography is quite adequate for identification of mature follicles, but its poorer resolution can miss smaller follicles. Endovaginal sonography provides considerable enhancement in visualization of these smaller follicles, which may be implicated in hyperstimulation. When oocyte aspiration is not performed, it is prudent not to trigger ovulation if more than four mature or a total of nine mature and intermediate follicles appear, for fear of hyperstimulation.

Hyperstimulation is less of a concern in IVF, because the aspiration of follicular contents seems to protect against the severe complications of overstimulation. Nevertheless, visualization of small follicles is also important. Aspiration of immature oocytes results in poorer fertilization rates and a higher chance of polyspermy. While a single leading follicle may be mature, others in the cohort may not be ready to be fertilized. It is probably a better idea to continue menotropin stimulation until most of the follicles have reached a mature size. Continuing the stimulation may sacrifice the leading follicle, but will more likely result in a greater number of fertilizable oocytes.

Endovaginal sonography is currently the preferred method for follicle identification. The major advantages of endovaginal sonography over abdominal scanning are the ability to visualize the ovaries without the need for bladder filling, the more precise visualization of small follicles, and the better resolution, allowing for identification of follicular contents. The increased patient comfort that results from scanning with an empty bladder is of very practical importance. Busy IVF programs often schedule ultrasound examination for a fixed time of the day. Furthermore, patients often travel long distances each morning to have their ultrasound scanning performed. Women undergoing IVF are not ill and would like to lessen the impact that IVF has upon their lifestyles. The ability to scan without preparation of bladder filling adds convenience and considerable comfort to the patient. Nero and colleagues found that patients who have undergone both abdominal and endovaginal scanning universally prefer endovaginal sonography.

In addition to the size of the follicle, the appearance of follicular contents on ultrasound can indicate follicular maturity. During the process of follicular growth, there is an accumulation of antral fluid within the antral space. At the same time, the layers of granulosa cell surrounding the oocyte differentiate into the cumulus oophorus and the corona radiata. The increase in thickness of the supporting cells surrounding the oocyte may be seen as the appearance of intrafollicular echoes. This information can not be well visualized transabdominally and is quite readily available endovaginally (Fig. 11–2).

Endometrial Assessment

Ultrasonic measurement of the endometrium may also prove to be a marker of oocyte maturity. The endometrium is easily visualized on ultrasonic examination of the pelvis, particularly with endovaginal scanning (Fig. 11–3). The endometrial echo is seen in the center of the myometrium and on longitudinal scanning appears as a triple stripe in the long axis of the uterus. Endometrial thickness is a function of the degree of estrogen stimulation and is correlated with the serum estradiol concentration. Patients with higher serum estradiol levels are more likely to implant embryos transferred into the endometrial cavity, possibly because of better endometrial development. The state of the endometrium on ultrasonic examination does not, however, correlate with success in in vitro fertilization. It seems that other factors, such as

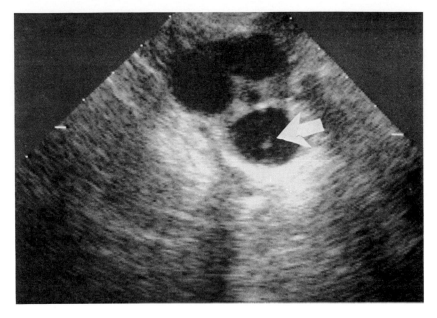

Fig. 11-2. Endovaginal view of ovaries following hCG administration. The arrow is pointing at a mass of cumulus cells. This follicle contained a mature oocyte.

the number and health of the embryos, supersede the endometrium as a predictor of successful outcome. Nevertheless, the endometrium can routinely be visualized when scanning is performed for follicular assessment. It is important to note its appearance as a clinical clue of the level of serum estradiol.

Once it is determined that follicular maturation has occurred, a triggering dose of human chorionic gonadotropins (hCG) is administered. This results in resumption of meiosis by the oocyte and follicular maturation that allows the oocyte to be fertilized. With resumption of meiosis, there is a loss of the germinal vesicle and expulsion of the polar body. Only oocytes that have achieved this level of maturity are fertilizable. These events require 34–38 hours in humans, and oocyte aspiration is scheduled for 36 hours after injection of hCG.

OOCYTE RETRIEVAL

Historical Background

The first oocyte retrieval in humans was performed in 1966 through a laparotomy. With further refinements of techniques,

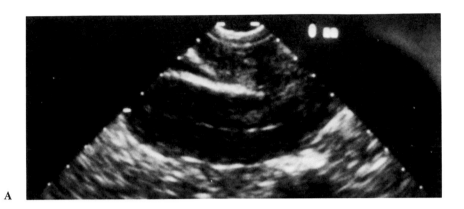

A

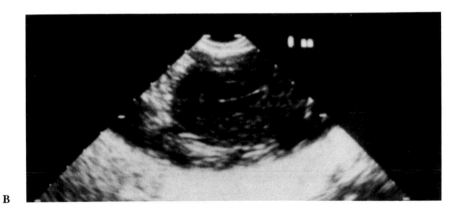

B

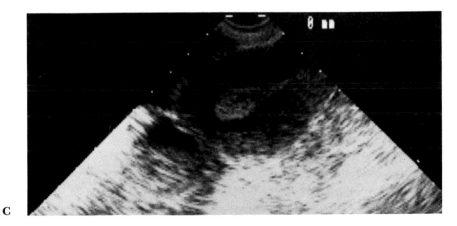

C

Fig. 11–3. Endovaginal view of the endometrium. (**A**) Early luteal phase. (**B**) Mid-luteal phase. (**C**) Late luteal phase.

Edwards and Steptoe successfully fertilized human oocytes recovered laparoscopically in 1977. Laparoscopy was the standard approach to oocyte retrieval for the first half decade in which in vitro fertilization matured as a therapy for infertility. While laparoscopy provided a safe and direct method for access to the follicles, several disadvantages soon appeared. First, many patients who require in vitro fertilization had pelvic adhesions, making it difficult to approach the ovary laparoscopically. Second, laparoscopy is a fairly invasive procedure that is not appropriate for patients who may require several attempts for a successful IVF cycle.

Improvements in ultrasound imaging have replaced laparoscopy with ultrasound guided retrieval as the preferred technique for oocyte retrieval. Ultrasound-guided follicular puncture can be performed with abdominal scanners that require a full bladder or with endovaginal scanners that do not have this requirement. Bladder filling is necessary in abdominal scanning because bowel usually overlies the ovaries, and gas contained within the intestinal lumen may obstruct visualization of the ovary. In addition, difficulties secondary to the long distance between the ovaries and the anterior abdominal wall can be overcome by acoustic enhancement through a fluid-filled bladder.

Just as the ultrasound transducer can be placed on the abdomen or in the vagina, the aspiration needle can also enter the abdomen through either route. Aspirations of oocytes can be performed through the anterior abdominal wall with an abdominal transducer or through the vagina with either an abdominal or a vaginal ultrasound transducer. One of the difficulties encountered with ultrasound-guided retrievals is proper spatial orientation. When the needle is not in the path of the ultrasound beam, it will not be visible, and control of needle movement is difficult. Therefore, both abdominal and vaginal ultrasound transducers are equipped with needle guides that directly couple the path of the needle to the plane of the ultrasound beam (Fig. 11–4).

The first ultrasound-guided aspiration of oocytes was performed transabdominally by Lenz and Lauritsen in Denmark. The approach used by the Danish team was transabdominal ultrasound with a transvesicle puncture. Initially the needle was not coupled to the transducer, but a needle guide improved the rate of oocyte recovery. Recovery rates in this series were 53%, which compares favorably with laparoscopically performed procedures. Transurethral and transvaginal approaches to the ovary using an abdominal transducer have also been used.

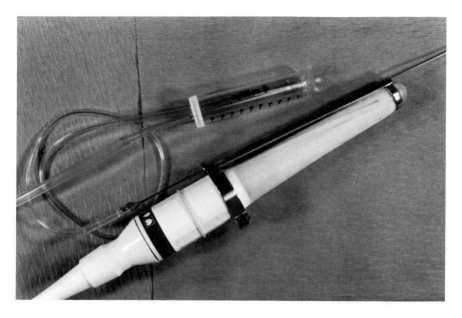

Fig. 11–4. The ultrasound transducer is draped with a condom. The needle guide with the needle attached is lined up with the path of the ultrasound beam. The De Lee trap is attached to the needle. Follicular fluid is collected in the De Lee trap and examined for the presence of an oocyte.

A major improvement in ultrasound retrieval occurred with the development of the endovaginal transducer. Ovaries that are surrounded by dense adhesions tend to be fixed to the cul-de-sac, a location that is most easily reached endovaginally. Prior to the development of endovaginal ultrasound, a surgical procedure was often necessary to fix the ovaries to the fundus of the uterus to allow access to the ovaries by laparoscopy. Ovarian fixation in preparation for IVF is no longer recommended and should not be performed. The most appropriate place for the ovary after laparotomy is its usual location, in the cul-de-sac.

The absence of bowel gas between the vaginal fornix and the ovaries allows the direct visualization of the ovaries without the need for a sonic window to enhance ultrasound transmission. In addition to the easier access to the ovaries in vaginal aspiration, the risks of bladder injury, hematuria, and infection that are associated with transvesical puncture are reduced. Endovaginal ultrasound-guided follicular punctures have resulted in oocyte retrieval rates of 60–75%, comparable to those obtained by laparoscopy.

Technique

The technique for endovaginal oocyte retrieval varies slightly from institution to institution. The transducer is draped with a sterile glove. It is important that this cover contain no materials that may be toxic to the oocyte and that all materials be tested with mouse embryos prior to their use in human IVF. Similarly, the coupling material that interfaces the transducer to the glove must be nontoxic. We use mineral oil for our sonic coupling, since many commercially available jellies are, in fact, toxic. The cover as well as the surgeon's gloves are copiously rinsed with sterile water. The vagina is similarly not prepped with toxic solutions, but rather is mechanically cleansed with saline. The needle guide is then placed on the transducer and the patient is given an intravenous sedative. We have found the combination of medazolam and fentanyl to result in adequate analgesia, and local anesthetics are unnecessary. An anesthesiologist is present for every case, so that deeper anesthesia can be administered if patient discomfort necessitates this.

The needle used for the aspiration has a 17-gauge outer diameter and is 11 inches long. It is important for ultrasound visualization of the needle that the tip be roughened to enhance reflection of the ultrasound beam. When this is done, the needle tip can be seen accurately, and precise placement of the needle can be accomplished (Fig. 11–5A,B). This is particularly important when the relationship of the major vessels of the pelvis is considered. The stimulated ovary lies immediately adjacent to the hypogastric artery and vein (Fig. 11-6). In order to prevent injury to the vessels, the tip of the needle must be visualized at all times. Another problem that can occur is misalignment of the needle with the ultrasound beam. It is important that the needle guide be secured to the transducer to prevent rotation from the proper axis. Misalignment of the needle guide will result in loss of visibility of the needle, with loss of precision.

The needle used for the oocyte retrieval has received a great deal of attention. If the inner diameter of the needle is too small, shearing off of the cumulus cells and possible damage to the oocytes will occur. In addition to the diameter of the needle, the texture of the inner lumen is important. A fine needle with an inner diameter of 18 gauge is more efficient than a coarse needle

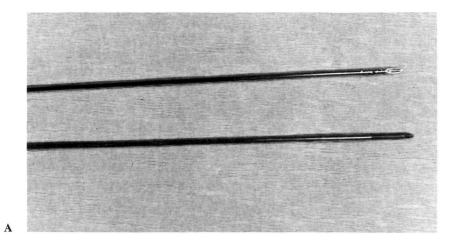

A

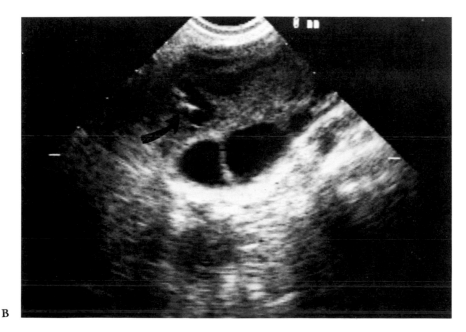

B

Fig. 11-5. (**A**) The aspiration needles are scored at their tips to aid enhanced echogenicity. (**B**) Endovaginal view of needle in a preovulatory follicle. The needle tip appears as a very bright echogenic structure (arrow).

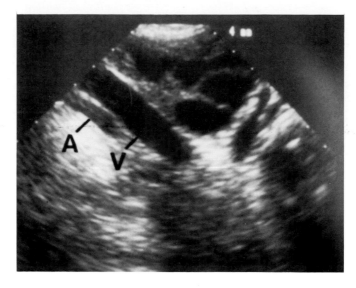

Fig. 11–6. The hypogastric artery (A) and vein (V) are demonstrated in close proximity to the stimulated ovary.

of 14 gauge in intact retrieval of the oocyte. Many programs coat their needles with Teflon for this purpose.

Anesthetic requirements differ with the various techniques available for oocyte retrieval. Laparoscopy is performed under general anesthesia, while ultrasound-guided aspirations have a lesser anesthetic requirement. Lenz performed transvesicle aspirations with local anesthesia and sedation, but the posterior bladder wall can not be anesthetized, and the transvesicle puncture is often quite painful. Regional anesthesia has been recommended by some authors for transvesicle oocyte recoveries. Endovaginal approaches to the ovary are less painful, and this procedure can be performed on an ambulatory basis with only intravenous sedation. Patients who have an endovaginal ultrasound aspiration under local anesthesia tolerate the procedure well. Hammarberg found that 90% of patients experienced some pain or no pain, while none described the retrieval as very painful. Premedication with a sedative and paracervical block was sufficient anaesthesia for 70% of patients, additional sedation was necessary for 20% of patients, and 10% of patients felt the procedure to be painful enough to require heavier anesthesia.

Dellenbach reported no major complications in over 800 endovaginal oocyte recoveries. Reports of pelvic infection following vaginal retrievals are unpublished, but there appears to be less than one infection for every 100 procedures performed. Because of the proximity of the hypogastric vessels to the ovary, care should be taken to avoid lacerations. The major vessels are easily visualized and avoided with endovaginal ultrasound scanning.

EMBRYO TRANSFER

A major drop in the success of IVF occurs after the transfer of the embryos. While 70–80% of oocytes aspirated will fertilize and cleave, only 20% of transferred embryos will implant. Although the process of embryo replacement is vital to the success of IVF, it is a blind procedure. It is hoped that ultrasound may improve success rates by permitting embryo replacement to be performed with guidance.

Routinely, embryo transfer is performed by the passage of a Teflon catheter loaded with embryos through the cervical os. The embryos are suspended in 90% serum to enhance stickiness. The column of embryos is placed between two smaller columns of media and air. The catheter is passed through the cervical os with the aid of a rigid guide. The tip is passed to the fundus of the uterus and is withdrawn approximately 1 cm, where the embryos are slowly expelled. Once the catheter is withdrawn, the contents are checked for the presence of residual embryos.

Retention of the embryos in the cervical canal is a problem encountered with embryo transfer. As the catheter passes through the cervix, cervical mucus sticks to the catheter, and embryos can become stuck to the mucus. As a result, embryos can be withdrawn along with the catheter. Schulman found that when the cervix is examined 15 minutes after transfer, fluid was noted in the os in 22% of cases. Poindexter et al. examined the cervical mucus in women who had had embryos transferred into the uterus and found that 17% of transferred embryos could be recovered from the cervix. As a result of these observations, transfers have been attempted under ultrasound guidance.

Ultrasound guidance has been utilized in two ways for embryo transfer. First, transabdominal ultrasound has been used to ensure that the transfer catheter is indeed in the endometrial cavity. As the catheter is guided through the cervix, a transabdominal ultrasound can identify the catheter tip to ensure proper fundal placement of the embryos. In cases in which cervical stenosis exists, passage of the embryo transfer catheter can be complicated by coiling in the cervical canal. This unfortunate complication could result in the expulsion of embryos into the cervical canal. In these cases ultrasound can be very helpful for confirming proper endometrial placement.

Alternatively, direct fundal transfer of embryos has been attempted. In these reports the transfer is performed transvaginally with a transfer catheter attached to the transducer, as in oocyte retrieval. The catheter is placed transfundally into the endometrial cavity. Once endometrial placement has been assured, the embryos are transferred. This technique has resulted in two pregnancies. While this technique holds promise for patients in whom cervical transfer is impossible, it does not achieve the pregnancy rate that routine cervical transfer can and is also considerably less comfortable for the patient. In cases in which difficulty with transcervical placement of the catheter is encountered, ultrasound can be a useful adjunct.

GIFT

Patients with normal Fallopian tubes can achieve higher pregnancy rates with in vivo fertilization in the tube. Asch and colleagues have demonstrated in couples with at least one normal Fallopian tube that transferring gametes into the ampullary portion of the tube (gamete intrafallopian transfer, or GIFT) achieved higher pregnancy rates than those of IVF. It is not entirely surprising that pregnancy rates are improved with in vivo fertilization procedures, since in vitro culture conditions attempt to simulate the Fallopian tube but cannot totally reproduce it.

GIFT is performed under general anesthesia with either a laparoscopy or a minilaparatomy. This is a major disadvantage to the patient, as the anesthetic requirements of laparoscopy are greater than for endovaginal ultrasound retrieval. Attempts to pass oocytes after endovaginal retrieval through the endometrial cavity under ultrasound guidance are under development. In this procedure, the oocyte retrieval is performed routinely via endovaginal retrieval. Once the oocytes have been identified, they are mixed with sperm in the transfer catheter. Under ultrasound guidance the catheter is passed into the tubal ostia and into the ampullary tube, where the gametes are expelled. The tubal ostia can be seen on endovaginal ultrasound, when air is injected into the endometrial cavity. A characteristic loss of resistance is also experienced when the tube is entered. Alternatively, the oocytes can be fertilized in vitro, and the resulting embryos can then, under endovaginal ultrasound guidance, be transferred into the Fallopian tube. Early attempts with this technique have been encouraging. In one series, one of five tubal embryo transfers performed endovaginally has achieved pregnancy.

SUMMARY

Ultrasound has several applications for IVF. First, ovulation induction could not properly be managed without follicular monitoring with ultrasound. Significant increase in patient comfort and improvement in resolution has made endovaginal ultrasound the preferred route for follicular monitoring. Second, oocyte aspiration is better tolerated and is safer when performed endovaginally. Oocyte aspiration can be performed in cases in which there are dense pelvic adhesions and ovarian access is difficult by laparoscopy. Third, transfer of the embryos into the endometrial cavity in difficult cases is more reliable when performed under ultrasound guidance. Finally, future developments may decrease the morbidity of gamete transfer by replacing laparoscopy with ultrasonographically guided transfers.

SUGGESTED READINGS

Asch RH, Balmaceda JP, Ellsworth, LR, Wong PC. Preliminary experiences with gamete intrafallopian transfer (GIFT). Fertil Steril 45:336, 1986.

Dellenbach P, Nisand I, Moreau L, Durand JL, Feger B, Plumere C, Gerlinger P. Update on experience with transvaginal method of oocyte retrieval. Abstracts Fifth World Congress on In Vitro Fertilization and Embryo Transfer, April 5, 1987, Norfolk P-013.

Diamond M, Wentz AC. Ovulation induction with human menopausal gonadotropins. Ob Gynecol Surv 41:480, 1986.

Fleischer AC, Herbert CM, Sacks GA, Wentz AC, Entman SS, James AE Jr. Sonography of the endometrium during conception and nonconception cycles of in vitro fertilization and embryo transfer. Feril Steril 46:442, 1986.

Hammarberg K, Enk L, Nilsson L, Wikland M. Oocyte retrieval under the guidance of a vaginal transducer: Evaluation of patient acceptance. Hum Reprod 2:487, 1987.

Jansen RPS, Anderson JC, Sutherland PD. Clinical pregnancy after nonoperative embryo transfer to the fallopian tubes. Presented at 35th annual meeting of Society for Gynecologic investigation. Baltimore, 1988, #421.

Laufer N, Grunfeld L, Garrissi GJ. Human in vitro fertilization. Present concepts and future aspects. In Seibel M (ed) Infertility. A Comprehensive Text. Appleton & Lange (in press).

Laufer N, Tarlatzis BC, Naftolin F. In vitro fertilization: State of the art. Semin Reprod Endo 2:197, 1984.

Lenz S, Lauritsen JG. Ultrasonographically guided percutaneous aspiration of human follicles under anaesthesia. A new method of collecting oocytes for in vitro fertilization. Fertil Steril 38:673, 1982.

Nero F, Diamond MP, Lavy G, Grunfeld L, Shapiro B, Russell JB, DeCherney AH. Patient survey of preferred method of oocyte recovery. Abstracts Fifth World Congress on In Vitro Fertilization and Embryo Transfer, April 5, 1987, Norfolk, pp 54.

Parsons JH, Bolton VN, Wilson L, Campbell S. Pregnancies following in vitro fertilization and ultrasonographically directed surgical embryo transfer by perurethral and transvaginal techniques. Fertil Steril 48:691, 1987.

Poindexter AN, Thompson DJ, Gibbons WE, Findley WE, Dodson MG, Young RL. Residual embryos in failed embryo transfer. Fertil Steril 46:262, 1986.

Rabinowitz R, Laufer N, Lewin A, Navot D, Bar I, Margalioth EJ, Schenker JJG. The value of ultrasonographic endometrial measurement in the prediction of pregnancy following in vitro fertilization. Fertil Steril 45:824, 1986.

Schulman JD. Delayed expulsion of transfer fluid after IVF/ET. Lancet 1:44, 1986.

Chapter 12

Incorporating Endovaginal Ultrasound Into the Practitioner's Examining Room

Previously, the use of ultrasound in the office by the Ob-Gyn practitioner has been mainly in the field of obstetrics. Currently, residency programs include training in ultrasound, but, as with any technical modality, those in practice have to make great effort to learn it through the varying postgraduate opportunities. Feeling secure in the skills required, concerns about liability, time required to perform the procedure properly, the size and expense of much of the equipment—all these factors have held many practioners back from incorporating ultrasound into their daily routine. Still others who do little or no obstetrics have never felt the need to get involved in sonography.

The new endovaginal probes will change much of this. When first introduced and marketed in this country, the emphasis was on infertililty. Virtually all in vitro fertilization clinics and many subspecialists in reproductive endocrinology realized the role of endovaginal ultrasound in follicle surveillance, ovulation induction, and oocyte retrieval (see Chapters 10 and 11). Still this represents a very small number of highly trained physicians. Endovaginal ultrasound, however, will undoubtedly result in an explosion of its utilization as part of the practitioner's daily routine. As a review let us examine some of the factors responsible for this.

PHYSICAL CONSIDERATIONS

This is the cornerstone of the utility of endovaginal ultrasound. Understanding this allows one to realize when endovaginal ultrasound is useful as well as when it may not be helpful. The endovaginal probes tend to be of higher frequency. They are also in closer proximity to the structure being imaged, resulting in very fine resolution even with high magnification. This means, however, a short range for the available focal zone. Thus endovaginal ultrasound is only helpful in the very near field. A minimally enlarged uterus may not entirely fit in one field of vision. This greatly limits the types of cases and therefore the types of patients for whom the endovaginal approach is appropriate.

The endovaginal scan is meant to be performed with an empty urinary bladder. Beginners will feel more secure with a small amount of urine in the bladder as a landmark (Fig. 12–1). As the bladder fills even partially, it will take up a majority of the available field of vision (Fig. 12–2). An empty urinary bladder saves time. It allows the procedure to be performed by the Gyn physician at the same time as the pelvic exam. This allows for instant clinical correlation of suspected diagnoses. The empty bladder is better tolerated by the patient. However, when the bladder is empty there is no sound enhancement, as is seen with traditional transabdominal scanning techniques. With the transabdominal technique, cases of increased fluid such as polyhydramnios in the fetus or pelvic ascites (Fig. 12–3) give the finest image production known to sonography. In addition, the empty urinary bladder means that loops of bowel are not pushed cephalad as they are in traditional transabdominal full bladder scanning.

In a Gyn office setting, the endovaginal scan is performed by the physician himself/herself at the time of the pelvic exam. Although it can still be done by a technician or nurse in a separate room, as is now done in many obstetrical situations, this will detract from some of its main advantages. The entire exam takes only 1–3 minutes to perform. This allows incorporation into the usual routine of a busy office day for appropriate patients.

It can truly be part of that patient's pelvic exam. The presence or absence of tenderness on pelvic exam is an important part of the synthesis of a correct differential diagnosis. The ability to image when palpating, the liberal use of the examiner's abdominal hand during endovaginal ultrasound, the ability to elicit tenderness if present with the probe while watching the structures in

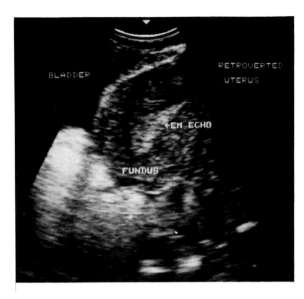

Fig. 12-1. Endovaginal scan showing a retroverted uterus in long axis. A small amount of urine is seen anteriorly in the bladder. The echogenic endometrial (EM) echo is labeled. The fundal region of the uterus is also labeled.

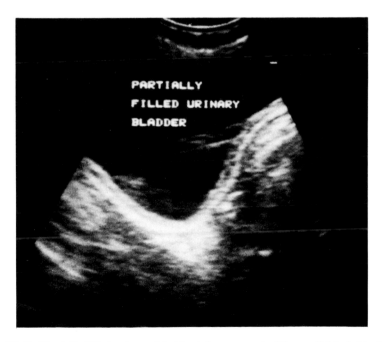

Fig. 12-2. Partially filled urinary bladder takes up most of the available field of vision because of the short focal zone of endovaginal probes. Ideally, endovaginal scanning is done with an empty or near empty urinary bladder.

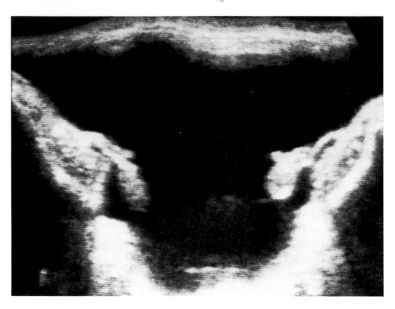

Fig. 12-3. Transabdominal pelvic scan of a patient with massive ascites. The sonolucent area anteriorly is ascites, not the urinary bladder. Note extraordinarily fine detail of ovaries and their suspensory structures from the pelvic side wall. Fluid in general enhances sound transmission and its presence always enhances image quality.

its path—these factors truly represent a marriage of the physical examination and the imaging modalities. Endovaginal ultrasound can introduce imaging into an appreciation of pelvic structures that was previously done "blindly," i.e., strictly by feel.

Currently, most companies make probes that can plug into "full service" ultrasound units. Most of these probes are mounted on handles. The future will see smaller base units that are truly more portable and less expensive, so hopefully someday every exam room will be equipped with one. The future may also see "finger probe tranducers" that can actually slip on the physician's finger and can be guided into the vaginal fornices by the pelvic hand during the bimanual examination.

INDICATIONS FOR OFFICE ENDOVAGINAL ULTRASOUND EXAM

In a relatively busy Ob-Gyn practice (about 15 to 18 patient visits per half day of office hours), it has been the author's experience that only certain patients will be appropriate candidates for endovaginal in-office ultrasound at the time of the pelvic exam. In a recent series, approximately one-fifth of the total volume of patient-visits represented routine second- or third-trimester obstetrical visits. These patients and any obstetrical scans that were indicated for them were excluded for the purpose of the study. Additionally, use of endovaginal scanning for infertility as a subspecialty situation was excluded.

Of the remaining routine office visits, about 18% had an indication for endovaginal scan at the time of their office visit while still in lithotomy position directly following a routine bimanual exam. Almost one-half of these were in the first trimester of pregnancy. Indications in this group included bleeding, size-dates discrepancy, pretermination surveillance, coexisting adnexal mass, and history of previous ectopic pregnancy. (The sonographic findings in such patients have been reviewed in previous chapters.) About one-quarter of the group scanned was done because of abdominal pelvic tenderness resulting in inadequate examination. Another one-quarter of the group scanned were done because of an adnexal mass or "fullness" of bimanual exam. Endovaginal ultrasound either confirmed an abnormal finding (Fig. 12–4) or corroborated normal pelvic findings (Fig. 12–5) in these cases.

A small number of patients were scanned for assorted other indications, including cervical region evaluation later in pregnancy, lost IUD (Fig. 12–6), and postoperative hysterectomy with pelvic fullness and elevated sedimentation rate (Fig. 12–7).

PROBE PREPARATION

Some equipment can be disinfected with a solution such as Cidex in between patients. Other users merely clean the shaft with alcohol. The endovaginal probe should be covered with either a specially fitted sterile sheath, the finger of an examining glove, or a commercially available condom. It should be pointed out that condoms are not sterile. In fact, they can be bought in bulk, arriving in large plastic bags. It appears, however, that individually foil-wrapped condoms that can be torn open under the patient's watchful eye helps to alleviate any patient anxiety concerning transmission of disease.

Whether a sheath, condom, or glove is used, the standard ultrasound coupling gel should be applied on the inside, and care

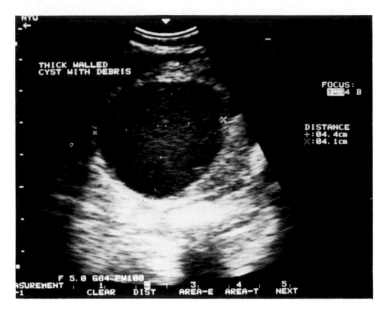

Fig. 12-4. Endovaginal scan of patient who on pelvic examination was felt to have a "fullness" in the adnexa. Scan here revealed a 4.4 × 4.1-cm cystic structure filled with debris (between cursors). This is compatible with hemorrhagic corpus luteum cyst or endometrioma. Follow-up scan in 6 weeks revealed increase in size. Surgical exploration confirmed endometrioma.

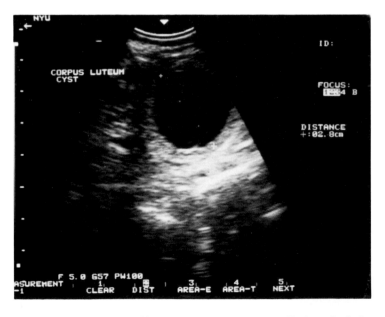

Fig. 12-5. Patient had "fullness" on bimanual examination. Endovaginal ultrasound exam here revealed a 2.8-cm unilocular cyst (between cursors) compatible with corpus luteum. Note how much of the available field of vision is taken up by a cyst even of this small size. Follow-up scan 4 weeks later revealed total resolution.

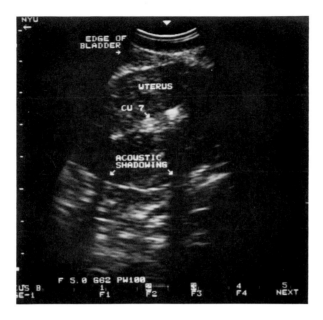

Fig. 12-6. Typical endovaginal appearance of copper 7 IUD (CU 7). Note the evidence of acoustic shadowing (arrows). A small amount of urine can be seen anteriorly in this long axis view of the uterus.

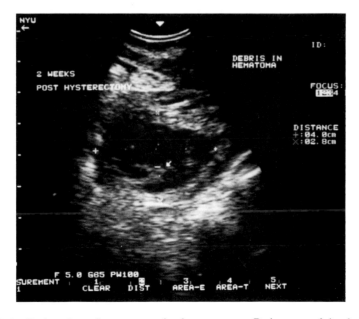

Fig. 12-7. Patient 2 weeks postoperative hysterectomy. Patient complained of pelvic pain and had elevated sedimentation rate and fullness on bimanual exam. Endovaginal scan here reveals poorly defined fluid collection with some solid debris (arrow). This represents a vaginal cuff hematoma that measured 4.0 × 2.8 cm. With antibiotic therapy, this collection spontaneously drained per vagina.

should be taken to avoid trapping any air bubble at the tip of the probe where it interfaces with the covering sheath. Prelubricated condoms are very messy to work with and should be avoided. A small amount of lubricating gel or mineral oil can be applied to the outside of the probe for insertion into the vagina. It should be noted that if an insemination of sperm is to follow the endovaginal ultrasound, some evidence suggests that certain gels may interfere with sperm motility.

PATIENT PREPARATION

The procedure should be explained to the patient. Often when the patient sees the transducer, a great deal of anxiety may ensue. It is helpful to explain that only a small portion of the probe is inserted into the vagina. Phrases like "smaller than a speculum" or "like a tampon at the end of a handle" can be most helpful. Occasionally, especially if the patient is in lithotomy position with draw sheet in place, attempts can be made to shield the actual probe from the patient's view.

It should be noted that an endovaginal ultrasound exam is similar to any other pelvic exam; therefore, consideration must be given to patient privacy, in terms of gown, draw sheet, and the need for a chaperone in the room as one would have for a routine pelvic examination. Obviously, the Gyn exam room will be equipped with a standard table capable of putting the patient in lithotomy position. This will enable full motion of the handle of the transducer even below the plane of the horizontal in an attempt to scan the entire pelvic region (Fig. 12–8). A flat examining table, as in a radiologic suite, would thus be disadvantageous in that the handle of the probe would be limited in the horizontal plane by the table. This can be overcome by placing the patient's buttocks on a thick foam rubber cushion or an inverted bedpan. (The latter is not particularly comfortable for an extended period of time.)

A small amount of Trendelenburg position, although helpful in abdominal ultrasound in trying to displace loops of bowel cephalad, should not be necessary for endovaginal scanning. Along these lines, however, it should be noted that because of the increased resolution due to the higher frequency and the close proximity to the pelvis, physiological amounts of fluid in the cul-

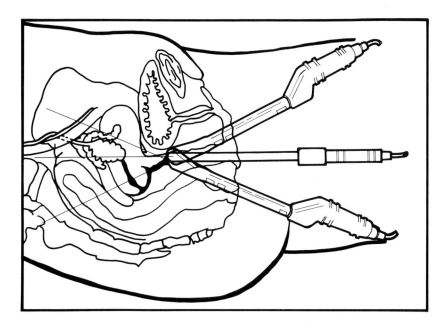

Fig. 12–8. Line drawing of the patient in a sagittal view. Note the various scanning angles produced by moving the transducer handle in a vertical fashion. A flat examining table will not permit the transducer handle to be placed beneath the horizontal plane of the table. Thus there is a need for the patient to either assume the lithotomy position or have her buttocks elevated from the table.

de-sac seem to appear more often in endopelvic scanning and should not be misconstrued as abnormal (Fig. 12–9). As with any other finding, this should be factored into the total exam and the clinical setting.

In general, nonobstetrician/gynecologists (radiologists, sonographers) do not perform a bimanual pelvic exam prior to the insertion of an endovaginal probe. They should be encouraged to overcome their reluctance to do so. As previously mentioned, endovaginal ultrasound is the marriage of palpation and imaging. The time has come for radiologists to learn the "laying on of hands." Prior suspicion of any mass, as well as the type of flexion of the uterine fundus and location of the cervix in the vagina, may enhance the study. However, even without prior pelvic exam, the

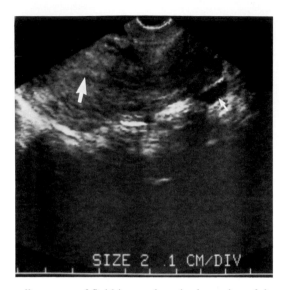

Fig. 12-9. A small amount of fluid is seen here in the region of the cul-de-sac (small arrow). The endometrial echo is outlined (large arrow). With higher resolution endovaginal equipment, physiological amounts of cul-de-sac fluid are often seen and should not be miscontrued as pathologic.

experienced sonographer will quickly find the pelvic structures to be studied and be able to identify other orientations with the pelvis.

Either the patient or the physician may insert the probe. Obstetricians/gynecologists will find that the probe can be inserted much like a speculum. A finger is placed in the posterior fornix of the vagina, and gentle pressure is exerted posteriorly. The vaginal area is much more sensitive anteriorly than posteriorly, and this depression of the posterior wall will allow for easy insertion of the probe. Many radiologists and technicians find it simpler to hand the probe to the patient, let her insert it herself (not unlike a tampon), and then allow the sonographer to continue the study.

The probe is inserted in the vagina either into the anterior or posterior fornix and then manipulated posteriorly or anteriorly and obliquely to the right or left in order to image recognizable anatomical structures. The beginner should be cautioned that occasionally the probe is placed too far into the vaginal fornices, and it is necessary to withdraw it slightly toward the introitus to bring the area of interest into the appropriate focal zone.

ORIENTATION

The vagina allows for limited mobility of the transducer. Certainly a midline sagittal (longitudinal) image can easily be produced. By turning the transducer handle 90° a coronal section may also be obtained. There is little latitude for moving the transducer in a stepwise longitudinal fashion to the right and left of midline. Rather, what one is doing in order to image the lateral adnexal structures is obtaining an oblique sagittal view to the patient's right and left (Fig. 12–10).

Traditional transabdominal pelvic scanning used multiple two-dimensional "tomograms" to mentally recreate three-dimensional anatomy. Our concept of "longitudinal" and "transverse" (Cartesian axis) is a throwback to static arm scanners producing images

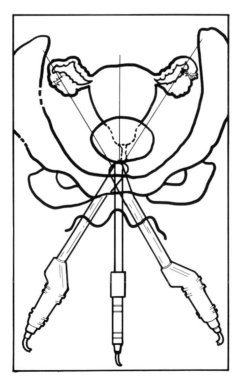

Fig. 12–10. The confines of the vagina do not allow for actual movement of the transducer in a longitudinal step-wise fashion. What one is in fact doing is angling the transducer in a sagittal oblique fashion in order to image the adnexal structures.

at 1 cm increments at right angles to each other. With the abdominal sector scanners that are currently in use today, views are still labeled as longitudinal or transverse. However, the operator is often angling the transducer head in a slightly oblique fashion such that still images are "frozen" to depict maximum recognizable anatomy.

In obstetrical scanning, one has long located an anatomical structure (i.e., fetal kidney or four-chambered view of the heart) regardless of transducer orientation. This is also true of endovaginal scanning. This is the basis for the concept of "anatomy-derived orientation." In endovaginal ultrasound, one looks for recognizable anatomy, such as the uterine fundus with recognizable endometrial echo (Fig. 12–11); an ovary overlying the iliac vessels (Fig. 12–12); or an early gestational sac displaying its typical trophoblastic decidual reaction with the uterus (see Fig. 4–2).

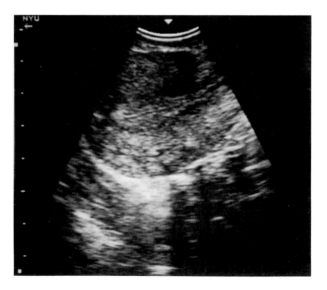

Fig. 12–11. "Anatomy-derived orientation" looks for a long axis view of the uterus that displays its endometrial echo. Thus the location of the anatomical structure supercedes the exact positioning of the transducer. The concepts of "longitudinal" and "transverse" lose the meaning they had with their origins in static scanning.

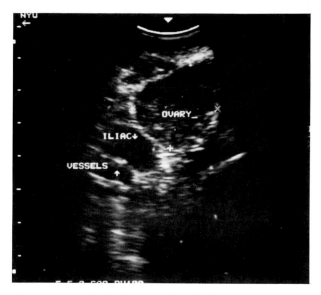

Fig. 12-12. "Anatomy-derived orientation" looks for an ovary seen often overlying the iliac vessels.

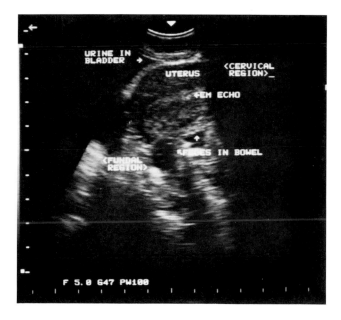

Fig. 12-13. Image labeling. This long axis view of the uterus demonstrates a small amount of urine anteriorly in the bladder as well as loops of bowel seen posterior to the uterus. The cervical and fundal regions as well as the endometrial echo are labeled.

Since the endovaginal scanning technique does not give a panoramic view of the pelvis when one is imaging an adnexa, it is imperative to label right or left. The uterus when imaged in a sagittal plane by convention will show the region of the cervix in the upper right-hand side of the screen, the fundus will be in the lower left-hand portion of the screen, and if there is a small amount of urine present in the bladder, this will be in the upper left-hand portion (Fig. 12–13).

PITFALLS AND PEARLS

Examination begins with location of the uterus in its longitudinal orientation. This is best done by identifying the endometrial echo or intrauterine gestation, if present. The ovaries are found by angling the transducer in an oblique sagittal fashion. Often they are seen overlying the iliac vessels, which can be identified by the pulsation of the smaller iliac artery.

Axiom Number 1

The more normal in appearance a gestation is, whether located inside or outside the uterus, the more likely it is to be visualized on ultrasound, regardless of technique employed (Fig. 12–14A–D).

Axiom Number 2

The more folliculogenesis contained within an ovary, the more likely it will be imaged with endovaginal scanning techniques (Fig. 12–15). The corollary to this is that the postmenopausal ovary without any folliculogenesis can be very difficult to image. It remains to be seen whether the lack of a finding in the postmenopausal state will be as reassuring as definitive identification of ovarian tissue that is normal in appearance.

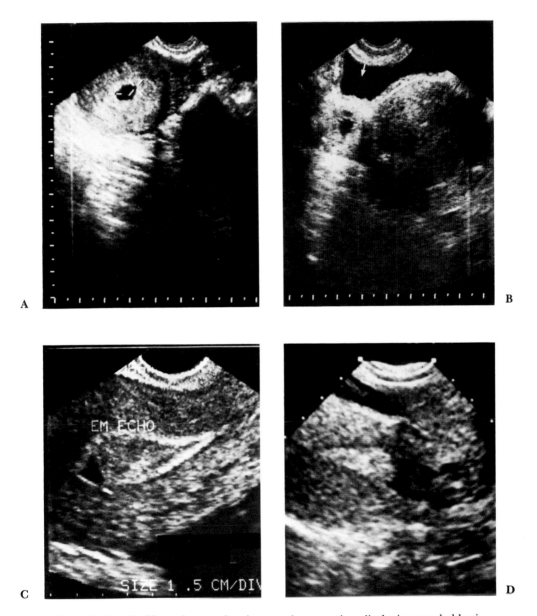

Fig. 12–14. (A) Normal-appearing intrauterine gestation displaying trophoblastic decidual reaction. **(B)** Normal-appearing gestational sac obviously extrauterine. Note small amount of urine anteriorly (arrow) in relation to the uterine fundus. **(C)** Endometrial (EM) echo in a "r/o ectopic." All one can say definitively is that this is not a normal intrauterine gestation. Previously referred to as a "decidual cast," this merely represents nondiagnostic endometrial findings (see **D**). **(D)** Endometrial echo of another patient who was "r/o ectopic." Curettage revealed intrauterine chorionic villi. Thus this patient had a missed abortion. Again all one can say definitively, based on this ultrasound scan, is that this is not a *normal* intrauterine pregnancy.

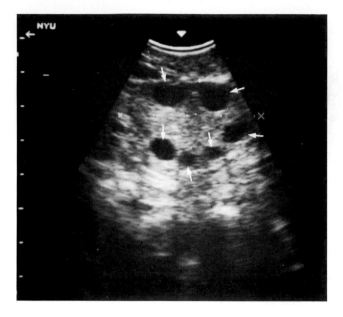

Fig. 12-15. Multiple small follicles (arrows) contained within this ovary allow for easier recognition ultrasonographically.

Axiom Number 3

Bowel is the bugaboo of ultrasound. Gas as well as solid and liquid fecal material produce bizarre complex echo patterns that are best recognized clinically by their motion (peristalsis) (Fig. 12-16). The corollary to this axiom, however, is that a focal ileus of bowel resulting in a lack of peristalsis can produce complex echoes that may not be readily identifiable as bowel in origin (Fig. 12-17).

Axiom Number 4

As one scans in a sagittal oblique fashion away from the uterus, the uterine vasculature may occasionally have an ovary-like appearance, which must be distinguished from the true adnexal structures (Fig. 12-18).

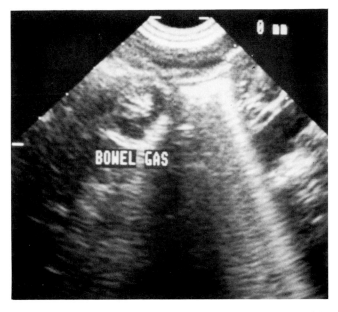

Fig. 12–16. Gas as well as solid and liquid fecal material produce bizarre complex echo patterns that are best recognized clinically by their peristalsis.

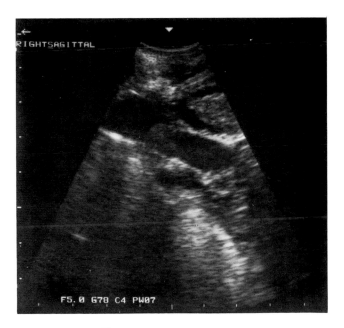

Fig. 12–17. A focal ileus, as seen here in a case of leaking ectopic pregnancy, can produce complex echoes that may not be readily identifiable as bowel in origin.

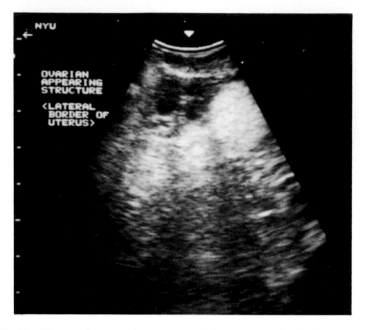

Fig. 12–18. The uterine vasculature scanned here in a sagittal oblique fashion can have an ovary-like appearance, which must be distinguished from the true adnexal structures.

SUMMARY

In summary, the future will see many endovaginal studies performed by obstetricians/gynecologists in the gynecologic examining room at the time of pelvic examination. This will allow the clinician instant correlation of the suspected findings in the bimanual exam, thus alleviating the necessity to refer the patient to a radiologic laboratory for evaluation. However, if the findings are at all in doubt, consultative ultrasound examination by the radiologist with transabdominal full bladder technique and/or adjunctive endovaginal study may be required to make a proper diagnosis. Knowing when to get consultation from someone more specialized is one major mark of a good physician in general. This is just as true for the Ob-Gyn practitioner who does endovaginal ultrasound in the office.

SUGGESTED READINGS

Goldstein SR. Early pregnancy ultrasound: A new look with the endovaginal probe. Contemp Ob Gyn 31:54, 1988.

Goldstein SR, et al. Very early pregnancy detection with endovaginal ultrasound. Obstet Gynecol (in press) 72:200–204, 1988.

Mendelson EB, Bohm-Velez M. Transvaginal sonography assessed early pregnancy. Diagn Imaging, November, 1987.

Schwimmer SR, Lebovic J. Transvaginal pelvic ultrasound. J Ultrasound Med 3:381–383, 1984.

Silva P, Platt L, Yee B. Transvaginal ultrasound in the infertility workup. Female Patient 12:14–24, 1987.

Timor-Tritsch IE, et al. Review of transvaginal ultrasonography. Ultrasound 6:1, 1988.

Vilaro M, et al. Endovaginal ultrasound: A technique for evaluation of non-follicular pelvic masses. Journal of the American Institute of Ultrasound in Medicine 6:697, 1987.

Wikland M, et al. Use of a vaginal transducer for ooycte retrieval in an IVF/ET program. J Clin Ultrasound 15:245, 1987.

Index